THE HOME HELP SERVICE

THE HOME HELP SERVICE

Margaret Dexter
and Wally Harbert

TAVISTOCK PUBLICATIONS

London and New York

Dedicated to the care,
concern, and commitment of
500,000 home helps, world-
wide

First published in 1983 by
Tavistock Publications Ltd
11 New Fetter Lane, London EC4P 4EE
Published in the USA by
Tavistock Publications
in association with Methuen, Inc.
733 Third Avenue, New York, NY 10017
© 1983 Margaret Dexter and Wally
Harbert
Typeset by Keyset Composition,
Colchester, and
printed in Great Britain by
Richard Clay (The Chaucer Press)
Bungay, Suffolk

British Library
Cataloguing in Publication Data

Dexter, Margaret
  The home help service.
  1. Visiting housekeepers—
     Great Britain
  I. Title   II. Harbert, Wally
  362.1′4′0941   HV687.5.G7

ISBN 0-422-78680-2
ISBN 0-422-78690-X Pbk

Contents

Preface

Like the police and the fire service, home helps are a well-known group of public servants. Most people have a mental image of the kind of work they do and the sort of people they are, but, as with most stereotypes, the image and the reality are often far apart. Furthermore, the role and tasks of home helps are changing; as services develop, the potential for further change becomes more evident, but progress is impeded by the out-of-date images of the service and what it can achieve held by the public and by staff in related services.

Placed as it is between the powerful professions of medicine, nursing, and social work, the home help service has struggled to find a realistic professional identity of its own. In the early 1970s it was reluctantly propelled from the protective skirts of the nursing and medical professions into the maelstrom of new social services authorities, where it was quickly dominated by the emerging profession of social work.

We have attempted to describe the way in which the service has developed in the past ninety years and how it has responded to changing needs to become an essential part of the total network of social care provided for many different client groups. We draw attention to its unused potential and to ways in which changes in organisation and training would equip the service to meet the challenges of the future. Descriptions of services outside the United Kingdom indicate the rich diversity of experience that can be drawn upon in planning future developments.

Whilst we have assembled material in a way that we think will be particularly helpful to organisers and home helps, we have been mindful that if it is to be effective the service must work in close collaboration with hospital staff, general practitioners, nurses, housing managers, social workers, occupational therapists, and a host of other specialist staff as well as voluntary organisations. We hope, therefore, that a wide range of professional carers will find this book of relevance to them, not only in their day-to-day contact with home helps and organisers, but also in planning future provision.

Because the home help service is an integral part of local authority provision it influences and is itself influenced by a great many local authority management, administrative, and professional staff, including officers employed in social services and social work departments, and staff with specialist skills in personnel, treasury, legal, and public relations departments. It is often these staff, who are employed 'outside' the home help service as traditionally defined, who have a decisive influence on new developments and on the ability of the service to change. We hope the book will be widely read by this important group of people.

Other readers who may find what we have written of value to them in their day-to-day work are councillors who make key decisions about the service and ordinary members of the public who may be among the 900,000 households in the United Kingdom receiving a home help in the course of a week. Finally, we hope that we will stimulate a greater interest in the service among academics, especially those concerned with social services education and training. For too long, training and research in the social services have been synonymous with social work as practised by field social workers and, more recently, residential staff. Few lecturers in universities or colleges have experience of home help provision and there has been little systematic study in academic institutions of its potential.

For convenience (and no other reason) we have adopted the convention of referring to the home help as 'she' and the client as 'he' throughout this book.

We would like to record our appreciation for the generous help afforded to us by many friends and colleagues. In particular, we wish to mention Melvyn Carlowe, Elizabeth Carnegy-Arbuthnott OBE, Sue Dowling, Andrew Edgington, Phyllis Harwood, Donald McDonald OBE, Laura Nepean-Gubbins, Doug Smyth, and Zena Williams.

We are grateful to the National HomeCaring Council of the United States and to Dr Sirkka-Liisa Kivela of Tampere University, Finland, for permission to describe in Chapter 5 specialist services in the United States and Finland.

Our grateful thanks go to our families for their forbearance.

Bristol, Avon   Margaret Dexter
January 1983   Wally Harbert

1 · A historical
perspective

The development of home help services in the western world is part of the social response to industrial and economic change. The pace and time-scale of change have varied from country to country, but across the world industrial progress has been accompanied by a significant shift in the status and role of the family and in the political aspirations of the working population. These changes have given rise to the development and expansion of health and social welfare services; although there are great variations in the ways in which services are provided in industrial countries there is, in nearly every western country, a clearly identifiable workforce that carries out home help functions. Just as the professions of medicine, nursing, and social work are internationally universal, so the home help service performs a discrete task and can claim recognition as a distinct discipline making its own unique contribution to social well-being.

There have been remarkable parallels in the ways in which home help services have emerged and developed in different countries. The same forces that influenced the birth and growth of the service in the United Kingdom have been at work in other countries and produced similar outcomes, but in this chapter we restrict our account of the history of the service to experience in the United Kingdom.

THE DEVELOPMENT OF DOMICILIARY CARE

The hundred years between 1750 and 1850 were characterised by growing industrialisation and a relentless transfer of population from the countryside to the towns, which were expanding rapidly. The social changes brought about by these processes were immense, representing perhaps the greatest peacetime social upheaval in the country's history.

The break-up of old communities and family support systems, coupled with recurrent problems of unemployment among a growing landless class, placed a great strain on the system of poor relief which had changed little since Elizabethan times. What had been predominantly an agrarian society based on reciprocal obligations between all classes was being replaced by an industrial society where community ties were loosened and the only effective obligation was the contract between master and servant. Parliament, in an attempt to reduce the burden of the poor rate, passed the Poor Law Amendment Act in 1834 severely limiting the scope of poor relief. The destitute were to be offered no support by the State in their own homes; those who were unable to provide for themselves were to be offered the workhouse where conditions should be more impoverished and unpleasant than those for the lowest paid worker.

The rapid growth of urban areas in the first half of the nineteenth century must be seen against the background of widespread ignorance regarding health hazards and personal hygiene. Impure water supplies, poor sanitation, jerry-built houses, and overcrowding led to high rates of infant mortality and constant epidemics. For many working men with families, wages were below subsistence level. Casual employment was common and spells of unemployment were a regular feature of town life throughout the century. There was no unemployment or supplementary benefit in times of hardship; the long dark shadow cast by the workhouse over the lives of the common people was as real, as sinister, and as strong a motivating force as that cast by the Church.

The Church and State were at one in seeking to uphold the sanctity of family life, but pursued this ideal by *laissez-faire* principles; that is to say, it was widely assumed that to provide financial assistance or to offer practical help to a family in distress would pauperise the family, making it less able to manage unaided. Although the word *pauperisation* has long since dropped out of common use, the sentiments embraced by it still find a place in current social and political argument and are important considerations in the provision of services. It has been replaced by more genteel epithets such as *disincentive* and *overdependency*, but the principle remains that in offering help to the needy there can be a danger of sapping self-reliance and encouraging dependence on outside help. In the nineteenth century the fear of *pauperisation* was so great that the workhouse was used as a deterrent. It was thought by many, including social reformers, that immense suffering and hardship were preferable to unregulated giving. It was commonly regarded as a mark of moral failure to 'go on the parish' and, for all the anxieties about creating dependency, once a family had demonstrated its moral unworthiness by seeking poor relief it was likely to suffer the most soul-destroying dependency of all – dependency on the rules and regulations of a closed institution.

It was against this background of political and religious beliefs about the inviolability and integrity of the family that changes were gradually wrought in society's expectations of the family and, indeed, in the role of the State as protector and defender of family life. The initiatives taken by charities to offer practical assistance to families in distress met with two counter-arguments: first, that by reducing individual responsibility charities would undermine family life and destroy the nation's moral fibre; secondly, that any assistance offered to families might have the effect of subsidising employers and keeping wages at an artificially low level. Attempts to promote legislation to improve social conditions were met with the same two arguments plus a third – that industry and trade could not survive if profits were to be diverted to help the poor. Any measure aimed at supporting or supplanting family life such as compulsory education or national insurance met with fierce opposition.

One area where significant improvements could be made in the life of the people, without challenging contemporary notions about the role of the family, concerned public health. The relationship between disease and the absence of pure water and adequate sewage disposal arrangements was established by the early years of the nineteenth century, and by mid-century strenuous efforts were being made to improve the sanitary conditions of towns. Surveys of houses occupied by the most wealthy in London showed that in many instances defective connection to the sewers meant that sewage sank into the soil under the basement.

In the care of the sick, the importance of what would now be considered simple, basic hygiene was beginning to be understood. Florence Nightingale's success in saving lives during the Crimean War was due more to her grasp of hygiene than to nursing skills as we understand them today. Hospitals were highly insanitary and increased the chances of infection and death. Poor living conditions in army barracks were shown to be more dangerous to life than some of the worst slums in the land.

There were many among the wealthy classes who were conscious of the extent and nature of poverty in society. By the 1850s it was becoming fashionable for ladies to engage in charitable work – described by Margaret Simey (1951 : 62) as feminine philanthropy. We are apt to scorn the 'Lady Bountiful' image evoked by wealthy ladies visiting the slums, but they were as much a product of their times as the belligerent young reformer is of ours. Indeed, it is difficult to judge which has made most use of the sufferings of the poor to meet his or her own personal needs. Social reform is an activity concerned with changing the balance of power and wealth and altering social relationships between different groups in the community. Inevitably it is based on the reformers' image of what is desirable. Lady Bountifuls undoubtedly alleviated much suffering in the nineteenth century and paved the way for the more organised and professional services that were to follow – in the same way that voluntary groups today help to spearhead new developments in social welfare services.

One organisation of charitable ladies described by Margaret Simey was the Liverpool Jewish Ladies' Benevolent Institution, formed in 1849 (1951 : 67). Like many similar organisations the institution would only help women who were adjudged to be deserving and of good character; where help was requested in connection with a confinement the woman concerned had to be married. To give help to those classified as undeserving was seen by Victorian society to be manifestly unjust and to encourage undesirable behaviour. Moreover, a charity that sought to help the undeserving would soon find it difficult to raise funds. In the twentieth century some charities have found a way around this by stressing that criminals, tramps, unmarried mothers, and alcoholics are victims of circumstances, or that early help will prevent further social evils. It was not, however, until the State became directly involved in the personal health and social services that the concept of equality of citizenship was established and assessment of need became a more important criterion for benefit than supposed moral worth.

Assistance was given by the Liverpool Jewish Ladies' Benevolent Institution with clothing and the loan of bedding, mainly in connection with confinement or short-term illness. The ladies soon found the task they had set themselves to be painful, unsavoury, and daunting. Margaret Simey reports that some of their number absented themselves due to 'their disinclination to remain in town during the unsanitary summer months' (1951 : 68). This conjures up images of foul-smelling alleys and courtyards, dank urine-saturated bedding, the smell of excreta throughout the house, and kitchens with cockroaches, beetles, bluebottles, mice, and rats. Such conditions would test the spirit of a modern trained and paid home help; it is little wonder that the voluntary ladies of Liverpool were often in deep despair. Nevertheless, such voluntary work was to become commonplace in towns and cities throughout the country; but the breakthrough in professionally based and paid domiciliary care came in 1859, also in Liverpool.

In that year William Rathbone, a wealthy merchant, was greatly impressed by the quality of the nursing afforded to his first wife during an illness which led to her death. He asked that the nurse should provide a similar service at his expense to a number of poor people in their own homes. Mr Rathbone's own account of the outcome, published in 1890 and quoted by Margaret Simey, cannot be bettered.

'As this was only an experiment, the nurse was not engaged for more than three months. But when one month was passed, she returned to her employer and entreated to be released from the engagement. Accustomed though she was to many forms of sickness and death, she was not able to endure the sight of the misery which she had encountered among the poor. But her employer persuaded her to persevere in her work, and pointed out to her how much of the evil which she had seen might be prevented, and that the satisfaction of abating it would in time be sure to reconcile her to the work. Thus reasoned with, the nurse persevered, and at the end of three months entirely corroborated the prediction. She found that she was able to do great and certain good, and the satisfaction of her achievements was so great that she begged to be allowed to devote herself entirely to nursing the poor in the place of nursing wealthy families.' (1951 : 71)

So impressed was William Rathbone with the outcome that he immediately sought to widen the service. Since there was a serious shortage of nurses with the skill he required, he consulted Florence Nightingale and on her advice set about establishing a training school in Liverpool. By 1865 eighteen districts in the city were covered by voluntary committees employing their own home nurses.

The concept of district nursing spread rapidly across the country. In 1887 Queen Victoria decided to devote money collected in celebration of her Jubilee to the development of district nursing and established the Queen Victoria Jubilee Institute for Nurses, to provide skilled nursing for the sick poor in their own homes. By 1902 nearly 500 branches had been formed throughout the country and the number of district nurses in London was said to exceed 100. Later the name was changed to the Queen's Institute of District Nursing.

Reports about home nursing in the early years stressed that it represented the highest and most exacting branch of the emerging profession. It carried great responsibilities with the fewest available resources. Home nurses found it necessary to cook, undertake housework, and manage children, in an effort to ensure that sick mothers could obtain adequate rest and relief. Ministering to the sick was of little value if there was no food in the house, if there was no heat, or if the risk of infection was increased by insanitary living conditions. The district nurse was, indeed, a Jill-of-all-trades and she undertook a range of duties now encompassed by district nurses, health visitors, social security staff, social workers, and home helps.

District nurses largely dealt with the practical problems surrounding illness in the home, but there was clearly potential for an educative function to be undertaken by trained nurses. Reformers recognised that improved hygiene in the home would prevent illness and reduce infant mortality. The Manchester and Salford Ladies' Sanitary Reform Association was formed to improve public awareness of the link between living conditions and disease in what was generally regarded to be the most unhealthy urban area in the United Kingdom. The aims of the association were 'to popularise sanitary knowledge, and to elevate the people physically, socially, morally, and religiously' (McCleary 1935). In 1862 the association developed a scheme employing paid staff to visit the poor, advising on ventilation, the prevention of infection, and the feeding and clothing of children; they distributed carbolic powder and urged parents to ensure that their children attended school regularly and that the whole family should be regular churchgoers. Although the first employees were not trained nurses – they were 'respectable working women' – this was the beginning of the health visiting service.

To Florence Nightingale goes the credit of persuading the first local authority to appoint a full-time trained health visitor. In 1892, as part of a health crusade in partnership with the Buckinghamshire County Council, she was responsible for organising practical advice to cottagers on ventilation, drainage, and general cleanliness.

In 1868 a new charitable body was formed – The London Association for the Prevention of Pauperisation and Crime. The main task that this new association set itself was to regulate charitable giving to avoid creating dependency among the poor. The following year Octavia Hill read a paper to the association entitled 'The Importance of Aiding the Poor without Alms-giving' and referred to the corrupting effect of indiscriminate charity. The association changed its name to the Charity Organisation Society and later to the Family Welfare Association, from which can be traced the origin of modern social work practice in this country.

The early district nurses and health visitors undertook many domestic and household duties that would now be regarded as the legitimate work of the home help service. They were often assisted by volunteers and by religious orders. The first recorded evidence of non-nursing personnel being recruited and paid to provide practical domestic assistance to the poor was in 1894. In that year Alice Modell helped to form the Sickroom Help Society in East London; the Jewish Board of Guardians, which had been co-ordinating almsgiving to the Jewish community in London since 1858, provided financial assistance for the society to appoint staff specifically to undertake household duties where the mother was confined or sick. During pregnancy mothers contributed a small weekly sum for the provision of service for two weeks during confinement. The home helps undertook housework, cooking, and the care of the children; they were not permitted to provide nursing care or to attend the patient in any way.

The country entered the Victorian era with a ban on what in modern jargon would be called 'State domiciliary services', while residential services underwent a rapid development. Although the workhouses, infirmaries, prisons, and mental institutions erected while Queen Victoria was on the throne remain with us today as a monument to social policies of a bygone age, by the time her reign ended a network of domiciliary services had been created by voluntary initiative, and the general principles of home nursing, health visiting, social work, and home help service had been established. Domiciliary care is not an invention of the twentieth century as commonly supposed – we have merely adapted and developed ideas and practices formulated when residential care was in its heyday.

THE RETREAT FROM 'LAISSEZ-FAIRE'

The development of domiciliary care in the latter part of the nineteenth century focused public attention on the evils of town life. For the bulk of the population life was so wretched that as services developed further light was shed on the miseries and privation suffered by large numbers of the population; the problems thus identified could no longer be ignored. Social researchers such as Charles Booth and Seebohm Rowntree painstakingly surveyed poor areas and showed statistically the extent of health and social deprivation. In his study of East London, Booth said:

'for the State to nurse the helpless and incompetent as we in our own families nurse the old, the young, and the sick, and provide for those who are not competent to provide for themselves – may seem an impossible undertaking, but nothing less than this will enable self-respecting labour to obtain its full remuneration and the nation its raised standard of life.'   (1889 : 165)

Rowntree (1901 : 206) established that in the poorest areas of York in 1899 one child in every four died before the age of twelve months; in one parish, one out of every three died in the first year of life. He examined the physique of large numbers of schoolchildren and demonstrated that in terms of weight, height, and general health children from poorer homes were significantly disadvantaged. He showed from army recruiting statistics (1901 : 217) that nearly 50 per cent of those applying for enlistment failed to reach the required standards of physical fitness. Nearly one-third of the rejected men did not achieve minimum requirements for weight, height, or chest measurements, which in the infantry were 8 st. 3 lb, 5 ft 3 in., and 33 in. respectively.

Although it was not possible to draw firm comparisons with the past, all the evidence pointed to the fact that the prevalent ideology which argued against State involvement in family life was not tenable in face of the new society which industrialisation and urban living had created. The development of the home help service runs parallel to attempts during the twentieth century to place greater responsibilities on government, both central and local, for the health and well-being of the population.

The high rate of neo-natal and infant mortality, together with accumulating evidence about the poor health and physique of children, focused public attention on midwifery services. In 1899 the infant mortality rate was the highest ever recorded. It was common for untrained women, known colloquially as 'handywomen', to offer their services during confinements for a small payment. They often possessed little knowledge and no skill. Frequently they provided the double duty of lying-in and laying-out and scratched a meagre living from the needs, fears, and prejudices of the poorest in the community.

In 1902 the Midwives Act created the Central Midwives Board to be the examining and supervising body of the midwifery profession. Its task was to ensure that only professionally trained and qualified persons attended women in childbirth. In the early years, the dearth of training facilities meant that a practising handywoman who could persuade a medical practitioner that she was responsible, could obtain a certificate from the board.

Maternity services remained largely in the hands of voluntary organisations until the second world war. At the beginning of the century charities often declined to assist single women. Mary Leslie, who trained to undertake the first examination set by the Central Midwives Board, described her experiences with the Newcastle Lying-in Hospital, a charitable organisation for married pregnant women, which, nevertheless, often delivered single girls at home. She explained:

'It was usual to find no water laid on and one had to find a kind relative to take the kettle down the street or alleyway to the nearest tap. That meant cold water and there was no coal fire. A search of our helpers probably found scraps of wood (some looked like skirting boards torn from the floor). Then there were no towels, not even old torn clothes, bits of which we could boil in the kettle if time allowed. In one case I took down a filthy old lace curtain from a window and rinsed it to wrap round the baby. Then the worst happened when the gas went out and no one had a penny to put in the slot . . . . All the time the smell in the room was nauseating; bugs, unwashed bodies and clothes, unswept floors with remains of meals rotting between the floorboards and all the time, too, neighbours coming in and being turned out, full of curiosity, sympathy and horrid tales about the lives of the neighbourhood.'

(1972 : 53)

The Liberal government of 1906 carried through many measures of reform to improve social conditions. The medical examination of school-children was introduced together with the provision of school meals. Pensions for the elderly, a medical insurance scheme, and the setting up of labour exchanges were also introduced in the early years of the century to tackle problems of ill health and poverty.

Whilst these developments represented new inroads into family responsibility there was a wariness about involvement in the homes of the poor. Domestic service was commonplace. The middle and upper classes relied on cheap labour to maintain their lifestyles. A Victorian hymn summed up the class consciousness of the time – 'The rich man in his castle, the poor man at his gate'. As an act of charity, affluent members of the community were prepared to support voluntary organisations that provided some domestic assistance to the sick poor who could demonstrate their worthiness; it was quite another matter for the upper and middle classes to pay higher taxes to provide the poor with the kind of domestic help which they themselves took for granted and which was the hallmark of social success. It would need a social revolution brought about by two world wars and universal women's suffrage for domestic help to the sick poor to be generally acceptable.

The first world war broke down many social barriers, particularly those relating to women's employment. Not only did women join the armed forces but many left their homes to work on farms and in munitions factories. They took jobs that had previously been reserved for men. These changes had a liberating influence on dress, behaviour, and attitudes. Women showed that they had a great deal to offer society as equals to men. They were less content to accept the long hours, drudgery, and poor pay of domestic service, or the rigid discipline that often accompanied it and the restrictions it placed on personal and social life. The growing emancipation of women opened up fresh employment opportunities and fostered a new political climate that led to greater State involvement in health and welfare matters. Ironically, however, it also created a resistance to domestic work, which was still associated with low social and economic status. The home help service is today trying to combat the image – and in some instances the reality – of an unskilled worker carrying out menial tasks with low pay and status.

In 1918 the Representation of the People Act completed the process of universal male suffrage started by the Reform Act of 1832 by giving the vote to all men over the age of 21; it also introduced votes for women over the age of 30. The Equal Franchise Act of 1928 gave the vote to women over 21 on equal terms with men. This legislation demonstrates the development of the concept of equal rights for men and women. Without the universal acceptance of such a concept it is doubtful whether State services for protecting children and supporting the family would have been achieved so soon.

The Maternity and Child Welfare Act of 1918 for the first time empowered local authorities to provide domestic help services in respect of maternity cases as part of a series of measures to safeguard the health of expectant mothers and young children. Government grants were made available to assist the development of services, and local authorities were required to appoint special maternity and child welfare committees.

Among the first local authorities to provide a domestic help service under the new Act was Bolton in 1919. In the following year the City of Birmingham followed suit, and gradually many large towns and cities started services or assisted voluntary organisations to do so. In 1920 a voluntary organisation, the Women's Service Bureau, ran a service in Liverpool, and in 1924 the City of Glasgow took over a voluntary service which had existed since before the first world war. By 1931 about one-third of health authorities were providing services, and in some areas these were organised on an agency basis by voluntary organisations.

In 1936 the powers of local authorities were widened to enable the service to be provided in any household where there were children under the age of 5. At the start of the second world war in 1939 about half of all local health authorities were providing a home help service directly or indirectly for home confinements. On the whole the service developed as part of the responsibilities of health visitors without specialist home help organisers. This arrangement continued in some areas until the 1970s.

The second world war brought about massive changes in social attitudes and once again stimulated public debate about the kind of society that should be built after the war. The years of economic depression between the wars had brought hardship and poverty to millions of people. It was hardly likely that those same millions would make personal sacrifices for the war effort unless they could be convinced that the future would be different. Throughout history, notions of idealism and patriotism have spurred on even mercenary soldiers to feats of bravery and endurance, but modern warfare is fought by conscripted armies, and the families they leave behind suffer great privations, not the least being brought about by enemy air attack. It is, therefore, necessary to create a vision of the future that will encourage the whole nation to put maximum effort into the war machine and that will sustain morale even when defeat seems imminent. Lloyd George found the right aphorism. 'What is our task?' he asked in a speech in 1918: 'to make Britain a fit country for heroes to live in'.

Plans were laid during the war years for the social and economic changes that were to be brought about as soon as circumstances permitted. The report prepared by Lord Beveridge (1942), setting out the broad framework for social policy, was keenly debated. To show its earnest intent the war cabinet and Parliament agreed legislation which brought about major changes in the educational system (Education Act 1944) and provided assistance to the disabled (The Disabled Persons Employment Act 1944). The momentum of social change which was set in motion during the early 1940s when the country was at war was to revolutionise social welfare services by the end of the decade.

But the war was making an immediate impact on family life, not least because increasing numbers of women were working in factories and on the land, leaving no one at home to care for members of the family who were ill or otherwise incapacitated. Absenteeism from factories was found to be largely caused by women who felt obliged to remain at home to care for sick relatives; similarly, servicemen and -women were seeking compassionate leave to care for their families. The demand for hospital beds could not be met and even minor epidemics of influenza put an intolerable strain on health services.

In November 1944 new powers were given to local authorities under the Defence Regulations. Authorities were empowered to establish domestic help services to assist households where there were problems due to illness or sudden emergency. In Circular 179/44 issued the following month the Ministry of Health outlined the circumstances in which help could be provided; they were

(a) where the housewife falls sick or must have an operation;
(b) where the wife is suddenly called away to see her husband in hospital and arrangements have to be made to look after the children;
(c) with elderly people who are infirm or one of whom suddenly falls ill;
(d) where several members are ill at the same time, e.g. during an influenza epidemic.

It is interesting to note that the circular automatically assumed that the husband and wife played traditional roles within the family, with the wife providing care and support whilst the husband was working or fighting; this concept was not seriously challenged in the provision of public services for another twenty-five years. The changes brought about in 1944 for the first time extended statutory powers to enable local authorities to provide services for groups other than expectant and nursing mothers, but there appears to have been little recognition of the role that might be played by home help services in caring on a long-term basis for the chronic sick.

By the end of the war in Europe nearly two-thirds of all welfare authorities in England and Wales had home help schemes operating under the wartime regulations, many being run in conjunction with voluntary organisations such as the Women's Voluntary Service. The home help service had a vital role to play in the development of health and welfare services. The country had experienced rapid social change and this was about to be reflected in the creation of new statutory institutions for the care of the needy.

WIDENING HORIZONS

The National Health Service Act of 1946 was a cornerstone of the massive change in social policy following the second world war. It established a comprehensive health service to be available to all members of the community. Section 29 empowered local health authorities to provide 'domestic help for households where such help is required owing to the presence of any person who is ill, lying-in, an expectant mother, mentally defective, aged or a child not over compulsory school age'. Authorities were authorised to recover charges for the service. The National Health Service Act brought together in one unified service the work previously undertaken for maternity cases under public health legislation and that for other cases under the statutory rules and orders of 1944; however, another twenty years were to pass before it became obligatory for local authorities to provide a home help service. Nevertheless, by 1957 all authorities were reported to be providing a service, although the extent and nature of the provision varied.

Money to expand public services was strictly limited in the years following the war. Not only was industry re-equipping to win back lost export markets and to compensate for the sale of overseas investments made necessary during the war, but bomb-shattered city centres were being rebuilt, and the housing stock, which had been neglected in the war years and had suffered greatly from the war in the air, needed a huge investment. Every branch of government was seeking an expansion of its activities to keep faith with promises made when the country was at war. Despite the circumstances the home help service began to grow steadily.

Although the number of full-time home helps fell slightly between 1949 and 1953, the overall number of home helps in the service rose by 66 per cent and the number of clients served increased by 40 per cent. In the immediate post-war years the home help workforce in the United Kingdom rapidly outstripped the combined number of health visitors,

Table 1   *Growth of the home help service in the United Kingdom 1949–53*

	1949	1953	percentage difference
England and Wales			
full-time home helps	3,967	3,341	−16
part-time	14,688	26,724	+82
number of clients served	140,000	199,000	+42
Scotland			
full-time home helps	569	780	+37
part-time	1,708	2,880	+69
number of clients served	16,000	17,500	+9
Northern Ireland			
full-time home helps	92	234	+154
part-time	96	1,023	+966
number of clients served	1,400	3,400	+143
grand totals for UK			
full-time home helps	4,628	4,355	−6
part-time home helps	16,492	30,627	+86
total of home helps	21,120	34,982	+66
number of clients served	157,400	219,900	+40

Source: The Home Help Organiser 5, 2 (1954).

home nurses, and midwives employed by local health authorities. By 1962 over 55,000 home helps were employed in England and Wales. The increase in the workforce was matched by an increase in the number of clients served, growing numbers of whom were elderly: in 1953, 58 per cent of the clients helped were elderly; by 1960 the proportion had risen to 75 per cent.

The Institute of Home Help Organisers has played an honourable part in stimulating creative ideas within the service and maintaining high standards. A group of organisers formed the National Association of Home Help Organisers in 1948 to promote the advancement and improvement of the service, to provide information, and to establish and maintain co-operation with other organisations. The chairmanship was held by Mrs Margaret Ritchie, MBE, home help organiser for the Westminster division of the London County Council, who became the first president of the institute when it replaced the association in 1954. The association became an institute with articles of association largely to strengthen the collective ability of organisers to influence central government in the matter of training. Successive governments were not prepared to provide the necessary funds to train home helps; unlike most other countries, efforts to improve training in the United Kingdom have been largely directed at the organising staff, and training for home helps has been left to *ad hoc* arrangements at local level.

The institute was not content to establish itself as a strong organisation in the United Kingdom. From the outset it forged links with overseas services and was a prime mover in establishing the International Council of Home Help Services. The National Association of Home Help Organisers held an international conference in May 1952 in London; thirty-five overseas delegates attended, representing twelve countries.

Several delegates from European countries took part in the institute's Oxford conference four years later. During the course of discussions it was agreed to establish an *ad hoc* committee to prepare a constitution for a permanent international organisation. The committee met in Brussels in 1957 and two years later an international conference was held in Wodschoten in the Netherlands to inaugurate the International Council of Home Help Services. National agencies representing home help services in fourteen countries became founder members. Miss E. Carnegy-Arbuthnott became president, a post she held with distinction for fourteen years.

Whilst the Institute of Home Help Organisers provided a forum for debate and a mechanism for exchanges of view between organisers, its members found it difficult to bring pressure to bear on local authority members. The service formed part of local authority public health departments which were headed by medical officers of health with many different responsibilities relating to the health of the community. Even senior organisers were of low status within health departments, and few were given opportunities to present their reports to health committees or to argue their cause with elected members. Clearly a national council drawing together representatives of all local authorities, including local councillors as well as home help organisers, would provide organisers with greater opportunities to influence policy-makers. Furthermore, the institute was not an appropriate organisation to represent the United Kingdom on the International Council; it did not employ home helps or provide services, nor did it have a co-ordinating role. The United Kingdom did not comply with the constitution of the International Council and a new organisation was required to regularise the position.

Thus in 1963 two stalwart members of the institute set about creating such a council, Miss E. Carnegy-Arbuthnott – later awarded an OBE – and Mrs Laura Nepean-Gubbins, a past president of the institute; they were well suited to the task. Miss Carnegy-Arbuthnott sent invitations to local authorities to attend the first meeting in Coventry, discreetly failing to disclose in the letter of invitation that she herself was employed as an organiser. Forty local authorities were represented at the first meeting, and the council was financed largely by one or two organisers for the first two years of its life; such was the dedication and sense of purpose of organisers. In 1979 the National Council of Home Help Services had ninety-five United Kingdom local authorities in membership and had established a reputation for its national conferences and its surveys of home help services.

2 · Social care in
a changing world

THE BASIS OF SOCIAL CARE

A distinguishing feature of the human species throughout history is that he has created a network of obligations by kinship and neighbourhood enabling dependent persons to rely on a measure of support from those around them. Mostly instinctive and informal mechanisms have been at work whereby families or the wider tribe have defended themselves against outsiders and mutually shared tasks which meet basic physical needs for food, shelter, and warmth. Dependent groups such as children, the elderly, and the sick have been cared for by the wider group. Without shared responsibilities and a willingness for the strong to help the weak, mankind could not survive.

With the development of civilisation the obligation of the community to care for its dependent members became more formalised. In medieval times the Church and the landed gentry accepted some responsibilities towards the deserving poor, although the mentally ill and confused were commonly punished along with criminals and beggars because their behaviour appeared to threaten the foundations of society. A lack of understanding also extended into the realms of physical ill-health, where malnutrition and disease took a terrible toll of human life due to ignorance about simple rules of diet, sanitation, and personal cleanliness.

While feudal lords were all-powerful, the system of mutual obligations which were integral to the social and economic system was seen to be sufficient, but the growth of trade and manufacturing industry created a new society in which those who suffered pestilence, famine, or unemployment had no recourse. The Poor Law introduced the concept of State responsibility.

In western society the growth of industrialisation in the eighteenth and nineteenth centuries brought swift and dramatic changes, as described in Chapter 1. The social philosophies of a feudal society, primarily based on the productivity of land, could not cope with the changing situation; new systems had to be developed and new networks of obligation evolved to provide the nurturing and the care that was needed. The transition was painful. Disease and death stalked the industrial towns of western Europe on such a scale that neither Church nor State could respond effectively.

Two powerful resources then became available which, combined with the desire of the human race to eradicate disease and suffering, began to shape the notion that the State must accept fundamental responsibility for the care of its citizens. The first resource was knowledge – knowledge about the causes of disease, its prevention and effective treatment; the second was the growing wealth of industrial countries, coupled with the popular wish, expressed through the electoral system, for that wealth to be distributed to ensure that dependent groups such as children, the sick, the unemployed, and the elderly received State help.

The twentieth century has seen a steady development of health and social welfare services in all western industrialised countries in response to popular electoral pressure. As hunger and disease have receded, succeeding generations have been freed from considerations about how to ensure physical survival, and they have devoted increasing energies to improving the quality of life for those around them. Improvements in public services such as health, education, social security, and social welfare have not diminished the pressure for further development. Improved services become the new platform from which the next generation argues for more provision. As the supply of services increases to meet demand, so higher expectations are aroused and the gap between supply and demand remains constant or even widens.

Andersen has described how improved material well-being was made possible only by separating production from the household and the family, and that this change inevitably weakened the family. He goes on to suggest that unless western society had been able to create new social institutions to assume some functions formerly undertaken by the family, the resultant social conflict would have prevented the process of industrialisation. He concludes: 'Some countries where industrialisation has not been followed by the development of welfare systems have, in fact, experienced brutal tensions and conflicts. Some nations in South America are illustrative examples of this' (1981 : 3).

It is clear that expectations about future growth and public provision cannot be fulfilled. Until the middle of the twentieth century industrial growth was thought to be synonymous in western countries with increasing wealth, but now it may be necessary to mark time while the Third World catches up; in any case, the sheer pace of technological change and our imperfect understanding of how to manage a diverse, dynamic, and world-wide economic system have produced high inflation and large-scale unemployment in western countries. In a different social and economic climate to that which has moulded social aspirations in the past, future generations may be less inclined to the belief that annual incremental growth in private consumption and public services are inviolable gifts from God.

The family and the immediate community continue to play a vital role in the care and support of dependent persons, but that role is now shared with the State. In the provision of income maintenance the State has specific and clear legal responsibilities towards the individual in most western countries. It also has specific, although less clearly defined, responsibilities in relation to the education of the young, health care, and housing. In the field of social welfare, the dividing line between individual and family responsibilities on the one hand, and statutory care on the other, has proved less amenable to definition, and although statutory responsibilities have been laid upon public authorities, it is a matter of speculation and disputation as to how those responsibilities are executed.

The role of the family has undergone considerable change over the centuries. Once a necessary institution for personal survival, its responsibilities have been gradually eroded by other social institutions. Its essential roles continue to be the nurturing of children, meeting human needs for close and lasting personal relationships, and the provision of mutual care and support. Other modes of life have long been the subject of experiment and comment, and family breakdown is an increasing spectre of industrial life, but marriage has never been more popular. The stresses and strains that a modern industrial society places on individuals appear to be such that we are propelled towards close personal ties even though they often fail to provide the satisfactions we crave.

The concept of a society in which there is no sense of personal and mutual responsibility between individuals is alien to all human experience through the ages. There will always be some people who do not fit the pattern – those who cannot cope with close personal relationships and those who, because of their circumstances, no longer form part of a family group that offers care and support. Nevertheless, it is important that in providing personal social services every effort is made to support any threads of mutual care that exist so that services enhance family life rather than destroy it. Social welfare services provided on any other basis will create more social problems than they can possibly solve.

In the remainder of this chapter we describe some of the social problems that exist for dependent groups and their families in western society, and suggest the role played by the home help service as part of the community's legitimate response to these problems. Throughout, we maintain the view that whatever legal obligations may be placed upon State services, the individual and his or her family, together with the immediate neighbourhood, must, to varying degrees, accept responsibility for social well-being. A State service that assumed no commitment to care by the community it served would be as soulless an enterprise as breaking stones in a prison yard and about as productive. Where that commitment is absent it is the first task of statutory carers to revive it. As love begets love, so compassionate and sensitive care can rekindle a sense of personal worth and belonging, without which human life has little purpose.

CONTEMPORARY SOCIETY

There is a remarkable similarity in the social organisation of countries in western Europe. From medieval times, similar pressures brought about by industrialisation, the growth of towns, religious and political movements, and improved medical care have interacted to create societies that have a great deal in common. The United States, and other countries largely populated by way of immigration from western Europe, also reveal similar social patterns.

At the turn of the century, life expectancy for boys at birth in six western European countries ranged from 42 years in Italy to 54 in Sweden (Havighurst 1978 : 17). By 1970 it varied between 68 years in Germany and 72 in Sweden. During nearly three-quarters of a century not only has life expectancy dramatically increased but the disparity between different countries has narrowed. Improvements in sanitation, in hygiene, in medical care, and the development of inoculation against disease in children has extended the life span of individuals. At the same time there has been a decline in the birth rate in most industrialised countries as families consciously control the number of their offspring. As a result of these changes the proportion of elderly people in the population has been steadily rising.

Changes in patterns of employment have meant a gradual loosening of ties between the family and extended kinship networks. When families were largely self-sufficient it was important to sustain close personal ties with a wide group of relatives who could provide mutual support in times of difficulty, but rising material standards and the development of social security and of State, health, and social welfare services have decreased dependence on the wider family. This has been accentuated by the growing mobility of families. It is not uncommon to find families dispersed over a wide area; in these circumstances, except in times of acute crisis, there is little likelihood of close mutual support when social care is needed.

The development of new housing estates in the United Kingdom between the wars and immediately following 1945 had the effect of splitting up old communities and separating different generations. In more recent years the gradual shift of population away from large urban centres has continued, but inevitably this means that it is predominantly the young and the economically active who move, leaving behind the elderly and the handicapped. Social and economic changes have therefore led to an increasingly elderly population which is more alone and isolated. Rising transport costs due to increased oil prices may reverse the trend: there is already evidence that some city centres are being revitalised by young families, but these are predominantly higher paid executives.

Describing the effect of demographic changes in Sweden, Karin Soder, Minister of Social Affairs, might well have been describing any western industrial society when she told the International Congress of Home Help Services in 1981:

'In earlier times the three-generation family was the normal type. The older members had a natural and unquestioned place in the community of the family; concern for the aged came equally naturally. There were also meaningful tasks for the elderly to perform. In the course of day-to-day relationships between the children and old people, the experience of the latter was absorbed by the young generation. Today this experience is wasted, with many old people living the last years of their lives in solitude.'

It is a matter of speculation whether prolonged economic recession will lead to a return of the three-generation family, and whether there is social and political pressure to create housing schemes that more readily permit a family to care for an ageing grandparent in an adjacent, self-contained unit.

At the turn of the century there were fewer than 5 million people in the United States over the age of 65. Now there are about 26 million and it is estimated by the social security administration that the number will reach 65 million by the year 2030. About 11 per cent of Americans are aged 65 or over; the proportion in Sweden is 16 per cent and in England and Wales 15 per cent. It has been necessary greatly to develop health care services for this age group. The over-65s, who are the largest users of health and personal social services, continue to rise rapidly in many countries, especially the United Kingdom and Sweden.

With advancing years there is a marked loss of physical mobility, and housing standards and income levels decline with age. Thus as social needs increase the capacity of the elderly to cope is reduced. About 30 per cent of all over-65s in England live alone, and this figure rises to 50 per cent for women over 85 (Hunt 1978 : 15). In Stockholm 50 per cent of all pensioners live alone.

Improvements in health care have also enabled more handicapped children to survive their early years. Whereas in former times parents could confidently expect to outlive a child with spina bifida, mongolism, or severe mental handicap, there is now no such certainty. Similarly, many survivors of traumatic accidents are being kept alive, thus increasing the number of people in the population requiring substantial and permanent personal care.

Social changes brought about by demographic factors are making it more difficult for the family to provide the full range of personal care required by dependent groups. These changes can best be summarised by quoting an eloquent passage from the Finer Report on one-parent families:

'There has been a silent revolution in marriage habits in Britain in the last two generations. In the past a significant proportion of women could never marry because the large scale emigration or wartime slaughter of men reduced the number of potential husbands. Since the end of the second world war the long persistent surplus of women in the marriageable age groups has disappeared; there are now more bachelors than spinsters; and women have acquired equality of opportunity to marry. The proportion of the population which marries has increased to the point at which marriage has become a universal institution which working class boys and girls enter at very young ages and will therefore experience for long durations. More and earlier marriage has not resulted in a return to the large family of Victorian days. There has been a sharp reduction in childlessness; there are fewer only children; and there has been a shift to families with two and three children. Fertility has been compressed so that three-quarters of all children are born within eight years of their mother's wedding. . . .

These changes have given women a new life. In the past motherhood was the whole life of most women. Today mothers have more than half

their active adult lives to lead after their youngest child has reached
school leaving age. One result has been a transformation in the
character and age structure of the female labour force upon which the
economy has been dependent for cheap labour ever since industrialisation. On the eve of the second world war the representative woman
worker was young and single doing a job between leaving school and
getting married. Now she is married, over 35 and with a grown up
family.'   (Finer 1974 : 62, 63)

The extent and significance of these social changes on the ability of
families to provide long-term care for dependent persons should not be
missed. The modern woman generally expects to determine her own
future and is often not prepared to sacrifice her aspirations for the
drudgery involved in providing basic caring services to members of the
extended family. Where she is willing to participate she is more likely to
expect the State to recognise her involvement and to accept some
responsibility.

The changing role of women has extended into the day-to-day minutiae
of family life. Increasingly the roles of men and women are inter-
changing. There is a greater sense of equality between marriage partners
and of shared responsibility for child rearing and household chores.
During confinement or when illness strikes down the mother it is
increasingly likely that the father can have time off work to care for the
family and that he has the capacity to manage. Nevertheless, rising
standards also make it likely that he will expect assistance from State
services.

Another consequence of the emancipation of women is the steady
increase in the number of one-parent families. A woman with dependent
children who is disaffected from her husband no longer needs to cling to
him for survival. As a single parent she is likely to suffer insecurity and
loss of income, although this is not inevitably so; she does, however, have
a more realistic choice than in earlier decades. During the nineteenth
century the most frequent cause of one-parent families was widowhood;
now it is marriage breakdown.

Information about the number of one-parent families is unreliable. It is
known that the number of divorces is rising and that many divorcees
subsequently re-marry. What is not known is the number of parents who
have informally separated and the number of divorcees who are co-
habiting. It is clear that many parents and children undergo the
experience of being part of a one-parent family, but often they remain in
this state for only short periods. *Table 2* compares information
gathered by the Finer Committee in 1971 with estimates made by the
Office of Population Censuses and Surveys for mid-1979.

Table 2 *Number of one-parent families in 1971 and 1979 ('000)*

	1971	1979
female		
single	90	140
married	190	200
widowed	120	110
divorced	120	310
male	100	100
total	620	860

Sources: Finer Report 1974 : 22, and *Hansard* 23 July 1981, col. 225.

All industrial societies report an increase in the number of divorces, particularly the USA and Denmark. In England and Wales the number of divorces rose from 28,800 in 1951 to 120,500 in 1975, representing an increase from a rate of 2.6 per 1,000 of the married population to 9.6. In France, numbers rose from an annual level of about 30,000 between 1953 and 1963 to about 90,000 in 1979. Several western countries have simplified divorce procedures in recent years.

The growing incidence of one-parent families, and the disruption it brings to family life, not only adds to demands on the personal social services, but makes it more difficult for families to provide informal care for the handicapped and the elderly.

Concern about the disadvantages suffered by ethnic minority groups is echoed in many parts of the world. The stresses and strains of family life for racial minorities, particularly those in substandard housing, can lead to low standards of health care, poor educational attainment, and poor employment prospects. These problems have been well documented in the United States, Great Britain, and France, but other western countries face similar problems, including parts of Scandinavia where Laplanders form a distinct and disadvantaged group. Social problems of this kind require a broadly based approach involving many government and voluntary agencies, but the home help service has a role to play in promoting appropriate standards of home care and relieving pressure on families under stress.

The World Health Organisation suggests that changes in family and community support systems and rising personal expectations of a consumer orientated society have led to a decrease in personal tolerance of stress (Baert 1981 : 1). The organisation has estimated that in thirty-two countries within its European region, 100,000 deaths occur each year by suicide, with ten times that number of attempted suicides. Consumption of alcohol doubled in Europe between 1950 and 1972, and there was a massive rise in alcohol-related problems such as alcoholism and road traffic accidents. One in five of Europe's population requires psychiatric help during the course of his or her life, and every third hospital bed is used for a patient suffering from a mental disorder. Drug abuse has become a large-scale international problem since the second world war, and the rise in crime rates is universal.

Increasing affluence is not reducing human problems – merely changing their nature. Infectious diseases and malnutrition are no longer prevalent in western society: they have been replaced by diseases relating to stress, by loneliness, and disturbed social relationships. It is a matter of judgement whether the families of one hundred years ago, whose members were largely illiterate and worked a twelve-hour day to ensure sheer physical survival, were less happy, fulfilled, and contented than many families of today whose members have a considerable measure of security and, as a consequence, find it difficult to develop purposeful relationships or achieve a sense of fulfilment.

CARE IN INSTITUTIONS

Industrialisation initially led to an increase in the number of dependent people cared for in large institutions. Throughout the western world in the nineteenth century, orphanages, prisons, infirmaries, and hospitals for the mentally disordered opened their doors to people who could not care for themselves. Life was often made unpleasant for the inmates to deter admission, and in the absence of community-based alternatives, large numbers of chronically sick people lived out their lives within the walls of drab and cheerless institutions.

We now know the debilitating effect of institutional care on the human personality. This has been defined by Russell Barton as 'institutional neurosis'. This he describes as 'a disease characterised by apathy, lack of initiative, loss of interest, especially in things of an impersonal nature, submissiveness, apparent inability to make plans for the future, lack of individuality, and sometimes a characteristic posture and gait' (1959 : 53). With the passage of time, changes in behaviour brought about by institutionalisation can overlay the symptoms which brought the patient into care, so that rehabilitation and discharge are made doubly difficult.

The smooth running of hospitals and residential homes requires residents to conform to at least some basic rules. Unfortunately it is easier for staff to manage an institution if they receive unquestioning obedience from their charges; at the same time, a lack of mental stimulation in an institution, coupled with infirmity or illness, can lead to residents becoming withdrawn, passive, and apathetic. Inadequate buildings, low staff ratios, and poor staff training increase the possibilities of institutional neurosis.

Long-stay care is often accompanied by a deterioration in personal habits and cleanliness. A lack of personal attention leads to a resigned acceptance of the situation, a loss of interest in surroundings, lethargy, and a willingness to accept instructions however unreasonable. In long-stay hospitals for the mentally disordered and in prisons it is common to see institutionalised inmates with drooped shoulders, head held forward, and hands held across the body; they shuffle along as though the joints in the lower part of their bodies are deformed; they are uncommunicative and isolated individuals who show little interest in the world around them and have no ambition to make a life for themselves outside the institution.

Although extremes of institutionalisation are well recognised and strenuous efforts are made to provide personal care and stimulation to overcome it, by its very nature life in any institution is restrictive and can easily sap individual initiative. This can sometimes be beneficial in the short term. Patients who are acutely ill may best be helped if they are allowed to lie quietly and are not expected to exert themselves. Their utter dependence on the nursing staff may be of therapeutic value. Nevertheless, as the acute phase passes it will be a necessary part of their rehabilitation for them to learn to make their own decisions and to exercise some influence on those around them.

Patients discharged from hospital often exhibit residual symptoms of institutionalisation. They frequently lack confidence to undertake simple tasks and deny that they are well enough to live at home. A planned approach to rehabilitation is needed involving the relatives and all the professional support concerned, including the home help service. But even those clients who do not enter hospital can show symptoms of institutionalisation if the care they receive at home is not carefully planned. Prolonged bed rest, in which the patient lives in enforced idleness, loses contact with personal friends, and is subject to impersonalised care, can produce what Asher described colourfully as 'a comatose vegetable existence in which, like a useless but carefully tended plant, the patient lies permanently in tranquil torpidity' (1947 : 967).

Institutional care leads to further hazards for certain categories of residents. It is common to find that lucid and rational old people become confused and rambling soon after admission to an elderly people's home or hospital, and that the mildly confused deteriorate further. Even a short period of stay, arranged to enable relatives to have a break, may lead to a marked deterioration of behaviour; if the resident becomes incoherent or incontinent it may prove impossible to return him or her home after a period of planned care. The change of surroundings and the tendency to confusion can lead to falls: for example, the old lady who gets up in the night, reaches out for the familiar bedside table not realising that she is in a strange bed, and as a consequence slips and falls, dislocating her hip or fracturing her femur. A medical complication following a fall is a common cause of death in the elderly who live in institutions, but large numbers of the elderly die soon after admission to homes and hospitals because they cannot adapt to the change in routine.

The development of high technology, the rising cost of health care in all industrial societies, and an awareness of the dis-benefits of institutional care have led to significant changes in hospital provision. Hospital admission is generally reserved now for those who need the expensive facilities of in-patient treatment; those patients who are untreatable are increasingly cared for elsewhere, and lengths of hospital stay are decreasing. Between 1972 and 1978 day surgery case attendances in England increased by 45 per cent, from 298,000 to 432,000 per year.

The number of mentally ill patients in European hospitals has fallen dramatically. From nearly 110,000 in 1969 numbers in England fell to 87,000 in 1975 and 78,000 in 1978. At the same time there has been a steady increase in the number of mentally ill patients treated in psychiatric units of district general hospitals, thus leading to a significant decline in the use of the old and remote mental illness hospitals. Day hospital places and outpatient attendances for mentally ill patients have steadily increased, and in 1978 about 4,500 mentally ill clients under the age of 65 in England were in receipt of a home help. The government has indicated (DHSS 1981a : 2) that 5,000 mentally ill patients in England could be discharged to the community if suitable care could be provided.

Rising public expectations about the quality of services have thrown into sharp relief the serious difficulties of trying to provide positive individual care for the chronically ill in large institutions. In the 1960s and 1970s a series of committees of enquiry were established in England and Wales to examine serious deficiencies that came to light in hospitals for the mentally ill and mentally subnormal. Despite increased expenditure on refurbishing old buildings, improvements in staff training, and reconsideration of management structures, long-stay institutions for the mentally disordered still give rise to concern. The problems will not be solved until the large old hospitals are replaced by small community-based units in which there is a greater emphasis on training and rehabilitation.

The movement away from large, remote institutions for the mentally disordered towards community-based care is a feature of all western societies during the past fifteen to twenty years. Professor Franco Basaglia has described his work in closing a psychiatric hospital in Trieste:

'After the second world war, Italian life and society were still rural in character but were changing rapidly into an industrialised society, and the formation of a working class after the war introduced many social changes. . . . Those of us working in asylums tried to change the relationship between patients and doctors to open up the hospitals and to organise a therapeutic community. This was not a new idea; we simply borrowed the English model. However, the background was totally different and it was difficult to introduce the English model into the very conservative situation in Italy.'   (1981 : 23)

Controversy still rages over the care of the mentally handicapped in Great Britain. Whilst the number in hospital has been steadily reducing – especially children under the age of 16 – services in the community have not been proportionately increased. Proposals put forward by the Jay Report (1979) for a radical reform of services for the mentally handicapped, to provide more family support and small-scale domestic units in the community, have been shelved through lack of finance, yet the government estimates that 15,000 – a third of all mentally handicapped patients in hospital in England – could be 'discharged from hospital immediately if appropriate services in the community were available' (DHSS 1981a : 2). In 1978 it was said that about 10,000 families with a mentally handicapped member received home help services in England, but this understates the provision because where elderly parents are caring for a mentally handicapped offspring home help assistance is categorised as being provided for the elderly.

Home care of the mentally handicapped can place a great strain on families: disturbed behaviour, hyperactivity, and incontinence are disrupting to family life, and even tasks like shopping and cleaning become major accomplishments when they are undertaken in company with a boisterous and unpredictable child or adult. Some seriously subnormal clients with added physical handicaps are now cared for at home because of improvements in special schooling and the provision of special care units where trained staff offer full care during normal working hours. Home help assistance for a few hours each week, together with opportunities for short-term care, is sometimes sufficient to enable parents to devote their full energies to the care of a severely handicapped child or adult who would otherwise require permanent hospital care.

Despite the significant rise in the number of very elderly people in industrialised countries which was noted earlier, specialist geriatric care has been slow to develop. In 1978 Brocklehurst (1978 : 165) suggested that geriatric services in Great Britain were twenty-five years in advance of any other country in the world, but the Department of Health and Social Security announced the previous year that targets for these services were not being reached, that staff ratios were too low, that consultant geriatricians had a low status among their medical colleagues, and that a lack of training for junior doctors was affecting recruitment to geriatric services (DHSS 1977). Geriatric medicine has been recognised as a specialty within the European Economic Community but does not have official recognition in all parts of the world.

Andersen (1981 : 6) refers to the fact that in many countries nearly half of all hospital beds are occupied by persons over the age of 65 despite a steady development of home care services. Until the number of elderly persons in the community began to rise dramatically little thought was given to the role of hospital care for the elderly, and all western countries are now examining their services to achieve a better balance.

Charlotte Nusberg (1981 : 206) explains that in the Netherlands concern over the high number of old people in institutions led to the creation of a central referral system in which every applicant for institutional care must undergo an assessment to determine the most appropriate level of care. She points out that

'it would be hard to find an industrialised country which is not expanding its community services in order to avert inappropriate institutionalisation . . . yet at the same time most countries are finding it necessary to expand the number of long term care beds because of the growing numbers of the very frail elderly. Generally, about 5% of the elderly population over 65 live in long term care institutions in both Europe and North America.'

The shift away from institutional care has not been confined to health services. As a policy it has been embraced enthusiastically by many pressure groups concerned with penal reform and by practitioners involved with the care of children. Unfortunately progress has been slow in these fields, but there has been a growth in community-based provision such as probation, prison aftercare, and community service orders for adult offenders, together with day care and family support in respect of children. The old established voluntary child-care organisations, such as Barnardo's and the Church of England Children's Society in Great Britain, are reducing their commitment to residential care and developing initiatives aimed at keeping children at home with their families. This often requires intensive family support in which the home help service plays a part.

The nurturing of children and their proper upbringing depends substantially on the personal qualities of the parents. All parents need assistance and advice from time to time but some, although capable of offering care and affection, easily become overwhelmed and lack basic household skills. There is a growing awareness of the serious injuries caused to children by violent and neglectful parents. Child abuse often occurs at times of personal stress, and it is frequently found that battering parents have had unsatisfactory childhood experiences leaving them unable to respond appropriately to the needs of their own children. The provision of a home help to ease a family through a crisis or in some cases to demonstrate good household management can enable a family to hold together. These were functions that were once carried out by the wider family and by near neighbours. The insular structure of industrial society makes it necessary for the State to intervene. The number of elderly people receiving care from the home help service is so high that it dwarfs the contribution being made in respect of families with children; nevertheless it is in this area that the service is likely to make a most important contribution in future.

INFORMAL CARERS

Care provided by families is informal, flexible, and personalised. When this care is replaced or supplemented by outside agencies there is an ever-present danger that the care will become formalised, inflexible, and bureaucratic. The family is multifunctional and at its best it provides integrated care. It is difficult for health and social welfare professionals to achieve the same degree of integration, since not only do professionals tend to limit their respective responsibilities to clearly defined tasks, they perform different tasks depending upon whether they are based in an institution, such as a hospital, or serve clients in the general community.

A physically handicapped person living at home may require help from a number of statutory and voluntary agencies. In the United Kingdom a need for financial support will be met by social security services; accommodation needs, including any special adaptations required to enhance independence, may be the joint responsibility of a housing and social services authority; nursing care may be provided by a home nurse; medical advice may be obtained from a general practitioner and also from a consultant physician based in a hospital; a physiotherapist, an occupational therapist, a volunteer visitor, and a day centre organiser may all contribute to the client's welfare; a social worker may assist him or her to make effective use of all these services. The scope for misunderstanding, lack of communication, and duplicated effort between all the professionals concerned is enormous. Unless positive attempts are made to effect a co-ordinated approach to service provision, the individual client is likely to feel misused.

The most serious problems of co-ordination occur when patients leave hospital, for, depending on their needs, they may require services from several agencies. Evidence on this subject discloses that communications between professionals based in hospital and their counterparts in the community are poor; even when they are good they are often not speedy enough to prevent serious problems arising for patients and their families immediately following discharge. The Continuing Care Project, a charitable body in England that has specialised in identifying the needs of discharged hospital patients and evaluating good discharge practices, has found that many patients return to cold, damp homes with no food; that there is often a long delay before medical, nursing, and home help services are commenced following discharge from hospital, and that caring relatives are often themselves frail or incapacitated and unable to provide the necessary help. One study of elderly patients discharged from hospital found that 9 per cent of principal caring persons had been admitted to hospital by the twenty-eighth day after the patient's discharge home (Continuing Care Project 1979b : 4).

There is universal agreement that hospitals exist primarily to treat patients who are ill, but there is considerable uncertainty and even controversy about their role in relation to the dying. As Holford (1973 : 4) has stated, terminal care

'would certainly not have seemed a controversial hospital function to Florence Nightingale. It is only with the development of the aggressive therapeutic attitude and the emphasis on active use of [hospital] beds that the death of a patient has come to be regarded as some kind of failure and his care a misuse of hospital capabilities. Perhaps the clock needs to be turned back a little.'

In recent years there has been a gradual increase in the proportion of deaths occurring in hospitals. It now stands at about 60 per cent in England. It is common for patients to be admitted to hospital within a few days of death. This probably arises because with an ageing population many people live alone or are isolated from those who might be able to provide care. Also, reductions in the death rates of children and young adults mean that death is no longer a common experience in families, and care of the dying is now more likely to be regarded as the province of experts. One consequence of the reluctance of relatives to care for the dying, and the ambivalence of some hospital staff, is the growth of the hospice movement. There are now about fifty hospices in England caring for terminally ill patients. The balance of medical opinion seems to support the view that the dying should be cared for at home provided conditions are suitable and that adequate supporting services are available. By their nature, domiciliary visits from general practitioners and home nurses are episodic; they bring support, advice, and treatment, but the patient and his or her relatives can often gain great support from the presence of a home help who is able to assist the household to function with a degree of normality during the last few days and weeks of a patient's life. Not only do relatives lack confidence in their ability to provide appropriate care, but they often have a real fear that support will not be forthcoming if difficulties arise; professional advice and assistance in the evening and at weekends is notoriously unreliable, and the increasing use of deputising services makes the family doctor less available than in former years. Improved night-sitting services can do much to reduce anxiety and enable relatives to provide the kind of care the patient needs. Unquestionably most patients would prefer to die at home, and many more relatives would be willing to shoulder the burden of caring for them if they could be assured of satisfactory practical support.

There is a growing awareness of the extent to which some families sacrifice a normal life in order to provide care for an infirm or disabled member. Inevitably, middle-aged women accept the greatest share of responsibility for dependent groups, but studies by the Continuing Care Project have shown that a considerable amount of care is undertaken by the elderly themselves. In one study of discharged elderly patients 49 per cent of the principal carers were themselves aged over 70 years (Continuing Care Project 1979a : 2). Wilkes (1973 : 31) found that 14 per cent of cancer patients dying at home in Sheffield were looked after by relatives who were themselves aged over 70 years. It is known that caring for sick relatives can be an unrewarding and burdensome task; there is evidence of marital breakdown, chronic misery, and loss of income brought about by the presence of unremitting care. Clearly well-developed home care services together with day attendance facilities and opportunities for short-term residential care can greatly assist relatives to provide effective care.

3 · Services in
the United Kingdom

For historical reasons, the legal basis of the service is different in England and Wales, Scotland, and Northern Ireland. Ministerial advice and guidance also varies since the component parts of the United Kingdom are represented at government level in different ways. Gathering facts about the personal social services is hazardous because government publications sometimes fail to make it clear whether they are describing services in the United Kingdom, Great Britain, England and Wales, or England alone. Recent figures about the provision of home help services are given in Appendix 1. Currently, about 130,000 home helps are employed in the United Kingdom.

A number of domiciliary services exist to improve and maintain the quality of life for families and individuals in need, enabling them to reach a higher level of functioning. It is difficult to embrace the tasks carried out by home helps within a short and universally acceptable definition, and, since there is an overlap of function with other domiciliary workers, there can be no clear differentiation between the tasks of home helps and other groups of staff employed in the public service. However, a list of tasks commonly undertaken in the United Kingdom is given in Appendix 2.

Home helps work primarily in the homes of clients, carrying out tasks that would normally be undertaken by members of the household, so that the client and his family can lead as normal a life as circumstances permit. Whilst the client's home is the focus of the service, some duties – like shopping, collecting pensions, and taking children to school – are performed elsewhere.

The service may be provided as part of a programme of care for a particular household, or it may have a rehabilitative and educative function in which the client is encouraged and enabled to accept greater responsibility for his own care. The style of work varies greatly depending on the assessment of need at the outset and the extent to which it is believed that rehabilitation is possible. In some instances both objectives are pursued in the same household. For example, the home help may prepare a meal for her client, deliberately encouraging the old lady herself to make the coffee to ensure that she remains active and continues to exercise her arthritic fingers. A third objective – control – is sometime evident as when a home help is responsible for children, the mentally handicapped, or very elderly, confused clients. These three aspects of the service – care, rehabilitation, and control – must be taken into account when assessing needs, when allocating home help time to a household, and when selecting the appropriate member of staff to provide assistance. Rehabilitation is more time-consuming than care. Preparing a meal for a client is a much simpler task than helping a disabled or depressed client to prepare one for himself. Control requires an approach that does not sap individual initiative or assault personal dignity. Different approaches are required depending on the need, which may vary with the passage of time.

No client is so devoid of ability as to be unable to perform some task for himself. The home help service must identify not just the limitations of clients but also the residual skills and resources they possess so that they are encouraged to use their capacities to the full. We all need to make decisions and to face challenges; a service that takes away the individual's self-respect and performs tasks he can undertake for himself saps initiative and deprives him of a sense of purpose. In our eagerness to provide care there is a danger of being very uncaring.

Tasks can further be divided into those that relate to domestic care and those that are of a more personal nature. Domestic care includes cooking, cleaning, mending, washing, and shopping. The second group, tasks of a personal nature, require some form of interaction between the home help and the client – washing, dressing, bathing, hairdressing, the provision of medication, feeding, and toileting all come into this category of work.

Services in the United Kingdom have been slow to develop personal caring functions and there is still some disagreement about the extent to which home helps can be expected to go beyond domestic duties. As long ago as 1949 the medical officer of health for the County of Kent disturbed delegates at a meeting of the Association of Home Help Organisers by saying that the service should confine itself to providing domestic help during normal working hours. A contemporary account of the con-

ference says: 'Members were plainly vexed. . . . There was no doubt from
the reaction of all present that the home help service is also providing
home care' (NAHHO 1949b : 2). In the same year at a conference held
by the National Institute of Houseworkers, the medical officer of health
for the City of Leicester said she felt that 'the ideal home help is a social
worker, more than just a domestic' (ibid. : 4). More than thirty years on
there is no doubt that the service provides more than domestic help, but
the question of the kind of training that should be made available to home
helps is only now being resolved.

It seems likely that services in Northern Ireland have concentrated
more on personal care tasks than has occurred elsewhere in the United
Kingdom. However, the Central Personal Social Services Advisory
Committee reported in 1976 that home helps had reservations about
whether certain tasks such as shaving, hairdressing, toileting, and
supervising medicines were appropriate functions for them (1976 : 6).
About 15 per cent of family practitioners in Northern Ireland who
responded to a questionnaire disagreed with home helps assisting with
washing, bathing, shaving, and hairdressing; about 10 per cent felt that
they should not assist in toileting clients. Clearly, without special training
it would be unwise for them to perform any of these tasks, but, in the
absence of other specialist services, unless the home help service finds a
way of responding to these needs the clients concerned will not receive a
service and their lives will be the poorer.

The essence of a good home help service is that it recruits, trains, and
equips its staff to undertake the appropriate tasks in respect of a range of
different needs, and that staff have the basic knowledge and capacity to
assess, in consultation with the clients and the organiser, the kind of tasks
to be performed and the extent to which personal caring tasks, or a
rehabilitative objective, should be pursued.

The personal relationship forged between home help and client is a
vital component in providing satisfactory care. Few people accept
incapacity gracefully, and help can represent a constant reminder to the
client of his inability to cope unaided. The trauma can be more readily
assuaged if the home help is a friendly, understanding person who takes
the trouble to listen to the client while he talks about his problems.

Depression and loneliness are central to the problems of a great many
clients receiving the service. The home help is often the key figure
standing between the client and total isolation. On occasions it can be
valuable for her to abandon domestic tasks altogether so that she can be
receptive to the strong feelings being expressed by the client. A survey by
Avon Social Services Department (1982 : 47) showed that 6.6 per cent of
all hours worked by home helps was spent in discussions with clients.

The home help must always remember that her workplace is the home of the client and that she must sometimes vary her approach to suit the particular circumstances that prevail. The Avon study found that for two-thirds of clients, no other person spent more time with them. The figure in Somerset was 43 per cent (Somerset Social Services Department 1980 : 79).

Unlike most other public employees engaged in domiciliary care, home helps spend many hours working with and for clients; their perspective and understanding of the way in which the client's household functions is therefore often quite different from those of other visitors to the household. The doctor, nurse, occupational therapist, social worker, and home help organiser carry out an examination and attempt to elicit answers to questions so that they can assess needs; the discussion is likely to be focused and highly concentrated; opportunities for observing how the client behaves are limited. The home help, on the other hand, is primarily concerned with enabling the client to respond to the physical and emotional needs of the day. She therefore sees the client in his unguarded moments and becomes aware of how he manages his life as opposed to how he says he manages it. Hers is a personal relationship as opposed to a professional one. The discussion in which she engages is not exclusively focused on the client and his needs but is likely to be more relaxed and reciprocal embracing her own personal life.

Unlike other official visitors she is likely to share the social and cultural background of the clients she serves. She invests more of her personality into her relationship with clients than is common with other domiciliary care staff, and to that extent she is seen by clients as a friend rather than a representative of an official agency. Audrey Hunt found that home helps believed that their clients mainly looked upon them as friends; for their part about 87 per cent of clients gave an enthusiastic *yes* when asked whether they liked their home help (Hunt 1970 : 293).

Home helps commonly gain considerable personal satisfaction from their work. They show a strong sense of personal loyalty to their clients, frequently going far beyond the call of duty to ensure that extra help is provided in times of particular need. It is known that home helps spend their own money on clients; they pay additional visits, they exchange gifts at Christmas and for birthdays; they undertake the kind of duties that an attentive son or daughter might undertake for an ageing parent. Audrey Hunt found that 15 per cent of all home helps undertook laundry work and nearly 14 per cent undertook ironing for clients in their own homes (p. 58).

Husbands are sometimes persuaded to assist by putting up shelves, mending fences, or tending the garden. In some parts of the country the additional voluntary work undertaken by paid home helps and their families probably exceeds the contribution of voluntary organisations to the care of the elderly. A survey by Avon Social Services Department in 1981 (1982 : 51) showed that 10 per cent of all clients received one or more extra visits from home helps within a seven-day period, while others were assisted by additional shopping trips and laundry work undertaken in the home help's own home. It was estimated that about 3,000 clients out of 11,000 assisted received additional unpaid assistance during the week.

The image of the service in the United Kingdom is still coloured by its origins. Domestic service has traditionally been regarded as a low-status occupation with poor pay and prospects. Although most home helps derive great satisfaction from the work and some continue in employment for many years, it is not regarded as an attractive career for younger women but rather as a convenient form of work for married women and for those who wish to work part time. Audrey Hunt found that the greatest incentive to leave another job to become a home help was a desire for shorter hours, and that new recruits were drawn predominantly from women in manual employment (1970 : 37). Just over half the home helps interviewed saw their work as primarily domestic rather than welfare, although about a quarter felt it was part domestic and part welfare (p. 62).

Observers of the service and organisers working within it who wish to enhance its status often stress the personal care content of the work. Hardly a conference goes by without a speaker saying that the service has changed 'from a cleaning to a caring role' or that home helps have 'taken the h out of charring'. It seems likely that the status afforded to the service by the public is lower than that of care assistants who work in homes for the elderly and handicapped, yet this latter group undertakes similar tasks and at the same time operates under much closer supervision and control. In the County of Avon, following a ballot of all home helps, the title was changed in 1980 to home care assistant and the service renamed the home care service. Whilst this has led to some initial confusion, the new name is very popular with staff and indeed with their husbands; since the change in title, staff turnover has been reduced and recruitment improved.

As with personal health and social welfare services generally, it is extremely difficult to measure or prove the effectiveness of home help services. Whether in a particular instance the service has improved the quality of life or effected rehabilitation is a subjective judgement, and the provision of a home help is usually one of a number of factors that have contributed to a successful outcome. It is significant, however, that all professional groups engaged in domiciliary care have a high regard for the service and constantly draw attention to the need for further development.

SPECIAL SCHEMES

The absence of clear policies and objectives for the service, the poor organisational structure, the lack of direction, the poor level of pay, and the paucity of formal staff training have created a service that concentrates on meeting the domestic needs of large numbers of elderly people on a routine basis. The average weekly allocation of hours – a little over three per week in most authorities – helps to sustain clients at home and to improve the quality of their lives, but services on such a scale can do little to assist those who are very frail and incapacitated and those with acute needs.

Local authorities that have sought to intensify their services, to ensure that they are real alternatives to institutional care, have found it necessary to establish special schemes which commonly include better training, better pay, more flexible and extended working hours, closer involvement with community health and hospital services, and an integrated approach with associated services such as meals-on-wheels, incontinent laundry services, night-sitters, and volunteer good neighbour schemes. Most specialist activities relate to the elderly, particularly the frail and confused, but modest schemes have been developed in different parts of the country concerned with the younger physically handicapped and the rehabilitation of families with neglectful parents.

From the earliest years the service has sought to meet urgent needs and to develop a capacity to respond flexibly. By 1949 at least three areas – Gloucester, Croydon, and Hornsea – had established night services (NAHHO 1949a : 3). In some authorities it was difficult to find home helps who were prepared to assist patients with tuberculosis, and relatives were being specially recruited to provide the service (NAHHO 1952 : 24). Special provision was made at that time for households that had become particularly dirty; often two or three home helps would be employed together in a team.

The Institute of Home Help Organisers reported in the autumn of 1954 that services had been widened to include night attendants for the chronic sick 'for whom hospital beds are neither available nor strictly essential' (IHHO 1954). Reference was made to the provision of home helps where patients were suffering from terminal cancer and from various crippling diseases. It was reported that services were being provided in the early morning and late afternoon to care for children whose mother was in hospital so that the father or other working relative could continue in employment. Emergency services, weekend working, and special residential home helps were all being provided to avoid the need to receive children into local authority care. Some authorities, including London, Herefordshire, and Rochdale, provided special home help services to multi-problem families, and in the institute's conference report for 1958 it is recorded that 'most of the organisers present had had at least a limited experience of dealing with problem families' (IHHO 1958b : 6).

Some services for multi-problem families involved special training for the staff concerned and enhanced payments. In Coventry, special home helps were recruited to work with families with low standards where there was a danger of the children requiring to be received into care. The role of the service was described as 'teaching, guiding and supporting the family, aiming not only to raise the household standards but also giving emotional support' (White 1975).

In practice a two-tier system of home helps has been slowly developing in many authorities whereby the normal service provides domestic assistance to large numbers of the elderly and handicapped while special staff, in association with other services, offer more intensive and special-ised care. The special staff are known variously as home aides, home care assistants, homemakers, home carers, the home help flying squad, domiciliary care assistants, home care aides, senior home helps, and social care home helps. Some are on enhanced rates of pay, some are covered by officer rates of pay and working conditions, and they are variously managed by home help organisers in collaboration with social workers and other staff.

It seems likely that in due course there will be attempts to rationalise the many different schemes that exist in the United Kingdom into a nationally agreed pattern. Trade union representatives in Northern Ireland suggested in 1976 that consideration should be given to establishing a number of different categories of home helps, each of which would have responsibilities for performing certain specialist duties and receive an appropriate rate of remuneration (Central Personal Social Services Advisory Committee 1976 : 8). The Northern Ireland Chaplains' Association indicated that a two-tiered system might be required whereby domestic duties were carried out by a home help while personal and medical care duties would be covered by a nursing auxiliary (p. 9).

A fresh impetus for the creation of new services in respect of the elderly occurred in the mid-1970s when it became clear that a substantial increase in the number of very elderly people in the population would not be accompanied by a commensurate increase in resources. The frail, the confused, and the severely handicapped would be required to remain in their own homes because no alternative provision would be available. It had taken twenty-five years for local authorities to develop residential services for the elderly to the extent that 2½ per cent of the over-65s were provided with accommodation, and there was little prospect of the rate of provision being accelerated. The government, professional organisations, and pressure groups were urging that care for the elderly in their own homes represented a better and more acceptable form of care than could be provided in elderly persons' homes and hospitals; with rapidly rising numbers in the very elderly age groups such a policy represented not merely a commitment to the development of community services to enable borderline clients to remain at home but a significant change in direction; it became necessary to organise home care for severely incapacitated clients for whom, previously, institutional care was the only available service.

Joint finance was a major instrument for change. This was a system introduced in England and Wales in 1976 whereby central government allocated specific funds to health authorities which were to be transferred to local authority social welfare services to meet the cost of jointly approved schemes of mutual benefit. There has been considerable flexibility in the rules surrounding joint finance, but the main component has been that approved social services revenue expenditure could be met by health authorities for a period of several years, with the local authority gradually absorbing the cost of ongoing schemes, so that after five or seven years the cost was met entirely from local authority funds.

At a time when local authority finances were under great pressure, joint finance represented the only opportunity of growth for some authorities. The availability of additional funds gave fresh impetus to joint planning between social services departments and health authorities, and prompted reviews of those services that were under the greatest pressure and where there was an overlap of function. It is, therefore, not surprising that schemes for developing home care services for the elderly featured in many plans that were formulated. Towards the end of the 1970s, particularly in 1978 and 1979, there was a mushrooming of home care services in England and Wales and the development of new initiatives associated with the home help service.

In a survey of new initiatives in the care of the elderly, the Personal Social Services Research Unit of the University of Kent has drawn attention to the fact that new developments in the home help service 'have attempted to shift the basis of the service from domestic to personal care' and in doing so many authorities have introduced similar schemes

(Ferlie 1980 : 3). An increase in personal care services is inevitably linked with an extension of evening and weekend working. Domestic work can mostly be carried out during normal working hours, but personal needs must be met as and when they arise. Thus specialist schemes tend to be very flexible and provide round-the-clock service as required. Many of these schemes are provided expressly to ease the transition from hospital to home. The home aide scheme at Bracknell in Berkshire and the homemaker service in Wirral were designed for this purpose. Derbyshire, Dorset, Gloucestershire, Surrey, and the London Borough of Barnet have developed services to facilitate early discharge from hospital. Schemes in Avon, Manchester, and Eastbourne have stressed the need for careful planning before the client leaves hospital, and in some cases home help organisers are located in hospitals to ensure that they play a full part in pre-discharge planning.

A full description of one specialist scheme will illustrate the kind of services that have been developed in many authorities in recent years.

'A pilot home aide scheme for the elderly was started in Avon in May 1978. A home aide organiser and ten full-time home aides were appointed to provide short term intensive support and practical help to clients within their own homes. The help provided was to be more intensive than that offered by the home help service under normal circumstances. Costs were met by joint financing.

A major aim of the service was to rehabilitate clients in their own homes so that conventional services could take over after a short period of intensive help. The two main categories of clients intended to be helped were firstly those ready for discharge from hospital but needing help to re-establish themselves at home, and secondly, clients who might need a place in hospital or residential accommodation, but who needed a period of professional assessment to determine the most appropriate form of care.

It was decided that at the time of referral there should be a strong likelihood that after six weeks the service could be withdrawn and replaced, if necessary, by other services. The level of support received by the client from family and friends was expected to continue. Home aides were provided free of charge, thus avoiding any discrepancy between the hours required and the hours that the client felt able to afford.

The home aide organiser and clerk were accommodated in their own office near the social work department in a hospital within the county. The home aides, who were appointed for their previous experience in one of the caring professions, regarded the hospital as their base and worked a five-day rota system over a seven-day week, providing cover to clients up to 24 hours a day. Upon appointment they received two weeks' intensive training in both health and social services authorities, including work on the wards of the hospital. This was followed at intervals by client care training.

Referrals to the home aide service were received by the organiser and a plan of care was arranged in consultation with all interested services. Where the client was awaiting hospital discharge, part of the plan entailed the home aide spending some time in the hospital to observe the programme of physiotherapy or occupational therapy, to talk to the ward sister regarding medication or to acquaint herself with the patient. The home aide was required to keep a written daily record of the client's condition to facilitate ongoing assessment.

The initial success of the scheme led to the creation of three further teams with a total of 50 home aides throughout the county. Analysis of the 513 clients who received a service in 1981 showed that the average weekly number of hours allocated to each client was 23½ although 22% received 30 hours or more. Nearly 10% of the clients received help at night. About two-thirds lived alone and, in the overwhelming number of cases, the home aide spent more time with the client than anyone from outside the household. Two-thirds of the clients were house-bound and over 40% had problems with incontinence.'

(Dexter 1981)

Oxfordshire social services department has pooled resources with a matching health authority to provide an integrated and comprehensive community service for the frail elderly in North Oxford and Abingdon (Quelsh 1981). The central aim of this project has been to draw together domestic and personal care duties and tasks usually associated with auxiliary nursing services. Home care assistants, after a period of one week's training, undertake duties including assisting clients to wash, dress, and bath; they also carry out the usual domestic duties of a home help. The home care assistants are required to work a split shift, the first shift normally beginning at 8 a.m., finishing at mid-morning or a little later; the second shift commences at about 6 p.m. and continues until 10 p.m.

Age Concern Liverpool has reported a scheme by which an intensive service of 'Aides for the elderly' replaces other domiciliary services such as home help and meals-on-wheels for the elderly mentally ill (Flynn 1982). Clients are provided with five hours of service each day, including weekends, by a rota of three part-time aides. The scheme is managed by a co-ordinator employed by Age Concern; a community psychiatric nurse has been made available by the health service.

The duties of the aides include the preparation of meals, dressing and undressing clients, escorting clients to the toilet, shopping, the management of money, laundry, household cleaning, the supervision of medication, liaison with relatives, neighbours and professional personnel, and, where possible, rehabilitative work. Because of the nature of the duties, applicants selected for training are paid, but the final selection of candidates does not take place until after the training period. A full evaluation is still awaited but indications after twelve months were encouraging. The cost of the scheme is met from joint financing monies.

Many local authorities have developed modest night-sitting services, often in conjunction with voluntary organisations. Sometimes, as in Doncaster and Birmingham, the night-sitting service is organised as an integral part of the home help service. Birmingham social services department also has two mobile night-watchers who can be contacted by radio; they work in conjunction with the department's emergency duty team of social workers and are, therefore, available to deal with crises.

The Northern Ireland Department of Health and Social Services in 1980 issued a circular (1/80) to each Health and Social Services Board encouraging them to consider how night-sitter services could be extended, either with assistance from voluntary organisations or by direct provision. Avon County Council is one of a number of local authorities developing an emergency service whereby a home help organiser is available to carry out assessments of need during the evenings and at weekends; she has a small team of home helps who can be assigned to emergency cases. Preliminary findings suggest that this enables suitable care to be provided during a period of stress and avoids the need to receive some old people and some children into residential care.

Social services authorities in the United Kingdom provide services for people in their own homes and in residential accommodation. Between these two distinctive forms of care lie sheltered housing, in which the client lives in a self-contained unit but has access to a resident warden who is available to deal with emergencies and carries out tasks that might be undertaken by a good neighbour. Such schemes are provided by voluntary organisations and by local authority housing committees. A frequent complaint about sheltered housing schemes is that the tenants are too infirm to live independently, that the overworked warden is unable to respond to the personal needs of so many frail and incapacitated people, and that hospitals and social services authorities are unable or unwilling to provide residential care for those tenants who are no longer suited to live in sheltered housing.

For their part, health and social services authorities have pointed out that sheltered housing is a very cost-effective way of providing care, and that with additional support it should be possible to retain more old people in this type of accommodation. This has led to the concept of *very sheltered housing* in which housing, health, and social services authorities join together to provide a package of services designed to ensure that sheltered housing is available to highly dependent groups.

Hampshire social services department, together with its matching health authority, arranged to offer more intensive services to sheltered housing schemes in 1976. Special arrangements were made for the provision of home helps, meals-on-wheels, short-term residential care, and intensive community nursing. In the same year Nottinghamshire social services department, with assistance from joint finance, introduced a pilot scheme in which sixty-three hours of care assistant time were made available to clients in each of two sheltered housing projects during a seven-day week. The work undertaken included personal care and domestic duties. Three further schemes were introduced the following year. Difficulties were encountered because the workload fluctuated: it was difficult to operate the service in a way that did not put unacceptable pressures on the care assistants at certain times and lead to an absence of sufficient work at others. Because of these difficulties and an overlap with the home help service, the scope of the service was extended beyond sheltered housing; care assistants are now based in the community and serve clients in sheltered housing and in ordinary accommodation.

A scheme provided jointly by the City of Bath and Avon social services department also recognises the need for flexibility in the use of home care staff. The social services department has guaranteed a measure of home help and other support from within existing resources. In addition, the social services committee is to make a capital contribution (from joint financing monies) towards the cost of construction of a new sheltered housing scheme to facilitate the provision of adequate support services. Features included in the design which are not normally part of sheltered housing schemes are a communal kitchen, which can be used for supplying meals to the elderly in the immediate neighbourhood; an enlarged community room, again for use by the local community; accommodation for a second warden; a central bathroom and a laundry. These features enable the scheme to offer valuable practical resources that assist in providing care to the severely incapacitated in the immediate vicinity, but because of the availability of these facilities it is also possible to provide a low-cost but effective home help service to those living within the sheltered housing scheme; home help provision will be free of charge to the tenants.

As long ago as 1965 the Ministry of Health urged local authorities in England to develop good neighbour schemes as a means of reducing pressure on the service (Circular 25/65); it was suggested that volunteers might tend fires, help with shopping, prepare meals, and help clients out of bed. Many local authorities have established close links between the home help service and groups of volunteers. In Buckinghamshire, West Sussex, Coventry, and Brent, joint finance has been used to enable home help organisers to appoint 'good neighbours' who provide assistance to clients for a weekly fee. This has proved a highly flexible and cost-effective way of meeting needs. A study by the London Boroughs Home Help Services Managers Group identified sixteen London boroughs in which home help organisers were responsible for good neighbour schemes (1978 : 43–4).

In order to respond to the increasing demands being made upon the service a study was undertaken by Avon social services department in 1978 to identify which tasks currently undertaken by home helps could be performed by a voluntary arm of the service. This revealed that approximately 1,000 clients could have all their needs met by volunteers, and that a further 1,500 could have part of their needs met in this way. This was from a total caseload of approximately 11,200 clients. Thus it was estimated that more than one in five clients visited by a home help could be provided with some assistance by a specially recruited and trained volunteer. It was estimated that the total hours per week that could be redeployed to the most needy clients as a result of the introduction of an alternative scheme throughout the county would be about 5,700 hours, equivalent to 142 full-time home helps.

A pilot scheme commenced in April 1981 in the Bath and Wansdyke districts of Avon. Organisers recruited volunteers – called home care associates – who were paid between £1 and £5 per week according to the nature of the task they performed and the time involved. Typically, home care associates worked for half-an-hour each day for their clients. The main task carried out was firelighting; in this area the traditional open grate was common because until recent years the main industry in the locality was coalmining and many of the elderly people continued to receive concessionary coal from the National Coal Board. The next most commonly performed task was shopping. Routine but vital tasks requiring a relatively small input of help were very suitable for this type of service. In most cases work was required to be done daily and the payment was designed to ensure a continuous commitment from the volunteer. This service was greatly appreciated by clients and their relatives and proved a useful addition to the home help service, releasing home help hours for redeployment elsewhere.

In future, the effectiveness of home help services will depend upon the extent to which facilities provided by statutory services such as health, housing, and social services can be mobilised to provide integrated packages of care for individual clients. The home help service has an important part to play in drawing together the full range of provision for the care of clients, and organisers will be required to increase the time and energy they now devote to collaboration with colleagues responsible for other services and for ensuring that full use is made of all forms of informal and voluntary care.

4 · Organisational arrangements in the United Kingdom

The home help service performs an important function in caring for people in great need. The extent to which the service meets the need presented is largely determined by the way in which the workforce is managed. This chapter considers changes in the organisation of social welfare services in the United Kingdom since 1948, describes the structure of local government and of social services departments, and discusses how policy is determined. Later chapters deal with charging policies, the assessment of client need, and employment legislation.

REORGANISATIONS

Although it created a comprehensive health service, the National Health Service Act of 1946 established three distinct units of administration separately managed and funded. Hospital services were administered by regional hospital boards and hospital management committees, which received finance from the national exchequer; family doctor, pharmaceutical, dental, and ophthalmic services were organised by local executive councils, also funded from central government; while community health services were provided by local authorities through health committees, which derived funds partly by way of government grant but also through local rates.

Differences in funding and organisation led to difficulties when patients were transferred between services. There was little incentive for local health authorities to provide services to keep people out of hospital.

In some areas hospitals found ingenious ways to persuade local health authorities to develop services. For example, the governors of the United Cambridge Hospitals came to an arrangement in the late 1940s whereby patients were discharged earlier than usual, and funds were provided from charitable endowments to enable the local authority to meet the cost of home help provision. In 1951 the County Councils Association announced that the scheme had been amended so that the hospital met the cost of the home help during the first week of the patient's discharge; the cost was shared between the hospital and the local authority for the second week, and the local authority became fully responsible thereafter (*Gazette Supplement* 1951 : 320).

Following the change from specific to block government grants in 1959, there was even less incentive for local health authorities to develop community services, since by doing so they increased their own financial commitment and at the same time reduced central government expenditure. The division of financial responsibility as between hospital care and the home help service has continued to this day, although since 1976 the provision of specific statutory funds has enabled the health service to allocate money to local authorities to develop services which are of mutual benefit.

The post-war development of health and social welfare services in Great Britain attracted considerable criticism due to problems that arose in co-ordinating provision. Central government was responsible for income maintenance through the national insurance scheme and national assistance – later supplementary benefit. At local level education and housing services employed welfare visitors. Local health authorities under medical officers of health were responsible for community health services, including mental health social work, but services for the elderly and handicapped covered by the National Assistance Act of 1948 were variously the responsibility of the medical officer of health or of separate local authority welfare departments. Services for deprived children were the responsibility of local authority children's committees created by the Children's Act of 1948.

Whilst great efforts were made to co-ordinate the work of these various organisations, it was inevitable that gaps would appear between services and that some overlap of provision would occur from time to time. Government circulars urged local authorities to establish co-ordinating machinery, but in the 1960s pressure was building up to reform the entire system. It was pointed out that trained social workers were employed in four or more departments of the same local authority, and that important services like day nursery care and the home help service were not easily available to staff in children's departments, yet they could play a significant part in rehabilitating families and avoiding the need to receive children into care.

The stimulus for radical change occurred in Scotland where the Kilbrandon Committee reported in 1964 on organisational changes in respect of services for children. The government took the view that the personal social services should be examined as a whole and it was not appropriate to isolate support for children from wider supporting services for the family and the community generally. A working group composed of representatives of central government, local authority associations, and independent advisers was created to consider the Kilbrandon proposal, and as a result a government white paper, *Social Work and the Community*, was issued in October 1966, recommending that social work departments should be established to cover the broad spectrum of social work and supporting services in Scotland. The proposals were enacted in the Social Work (Scotland) Act of 1968 and implemented the following year. Local government reorganisation in 1975 reduced the number of social work authorities to nine.

Meanwhile, in England and Wales the government established a committee at the end of 1965, under the chairmanship of Frederick Seebohm (now Lord Seebohm), to review the organisation and responsibilities of the local authority personal social services and to consider what changes should be brought about. The Seebohm Committee reported in 1968 on the need for organisational change within local authorities to bring together residential, day, and domiciliary social work services into a unified department separate from the health service. The committee saw the home help service as playing an important preventative and supportive function in helping to sustain dependent groups in the community. At the same time, the committee urged a significant expansion in the personal social services generally.

Home help organisers were not happy with the proposal that they should be transferred from the health service. They argued that the main reason for supplying a home help was medical rather than social, and that it was valuable for the service to be headed by a medical officer since he could effectively deal with complaints from general practitioners and hospital consultants. No doubt another strong reason was that organisers, although sadly neglected by the health service, could at least feel part of a service which, because of its medical context, attracted respect and a measure of status; transfer to a new department with uncertain aims and doubtful professionalism appeared to be a leap in the dark. Organisers had no reason to believe that their aspirations for improved training and recognition would be better served in social services departments; subsequent events have proved that they were right to be sceptical.

The Local Authority Social Services Act of 1970 implemented the main recommendations of the Seebohm Committee, and new social services departments came into existence in England and Wales on 1 April 1971. At about the same time significant changes were made in the provision of services. The Children and Young Persons Act of 1969 reformed the system for dealing with juvenile offenders, while the Chronically Sick and Disabled Persons Act of 1970 increased the range of duties of local authorities in respect of the disabled. A section of the Public Health and Health Services Act of 1968, placing a duty on local authorities in England and Wales to provide home help services, was brought into force in 1969, two years ahead of a similar change in Scotland. Local government reorganisation outside London in 1974 reduced the number of social services authorities in England and Wales to 116.

In Northern Ireland prior to 1973 home help services were provided by local authority welfare committees on the basis of a model scheme approved by the Northern Ireland Ministry of Health and Social Services. Reorganisation of the personal social services in Northern Ireland differed from that in the rest of the United Kingdom: social welfare and health services were combined into four area boards.

Reorganisation, and the expansionist philosophy of the time, led to significant developments in the personal social services. In the first year of the new Scottish departments the number of home helps increased by nearly 6 per cent, although in 23 of the 52 local authority areas the service continued to be administered by medical officers of health, since the Scottish Act did not compel the transfer of the service to the new departments. In England the number of full-time equivalent home helps rose from 29,700 in 1970 to 38,095 in 1973, an average annual increase of over 9 per cent. Reorganisation in Northern Ireland stimulated an increase in provision from 9,211 home helps in 1974 to 11,229 in 1975 – an increase of nearly 22 per cent – but the effect of public expenditure reductions lowered that figure to 10,447 in 1976.

The present functional boundaries between the national health service and social services provision were worked out for England and Wales in the late 1960s and early 1970s. The Seebohm Committee pressed strongly for unified social services authorities, whilst the Department of Health and Social Security, in a green paper on the national health service, set out the arguments for separating social and health care services. It said:

'the Government has decided that the services should be organised according to the main skills required to provide them rather than by any categorisation of primary user. Any alternative would involve the establishment of more than one local service deploying the same skill.

Broadly speaking, the decision is that the health authorities will be responsible for services where the primary skill needed is that of the health professions, while the local authorities will be responsible for services where the primary skill is social care or support. The scarce skills of professional people will be used to greatest advantage if those of each profession are marshalled and husbanded by one agency in each area. Moreover it will more often be possible to provide for users the advantages of continuity of care by one professional worker of any one discipline. Classification of services by skill will also help to enhance professional standards.'

(DHSS 1970 : 10)

Despite the poor pay and low status attaching to the task of home helps there is universal acclaim for the service. There are parallels with other forms of employment dominated by women – nursing and office cleaning are examples – where there is no shortage of praise, but an unwillingness to provide the kind of pay and working conditions that other groups of staff take for granted. But the sheer success of the home help service in caring for people in their own homes, and its inability to meet all demands, means that other professional groups would like to have more direct control over the service; this arises partly from a wish to be more closely associated with a successful enterprise, but also because different groups of staff have their own perceptions of priorities and tend to feel that if they controlled the service they would ensure that it was used more effectively to meet what they see as the most pressing needs.

The Harvard Davis Committee on the organisation of group practice urged in 1971 that home helps should be attached to group practices (Harvard Davis Report 1971 : 37). Gibson, a general practitioner with a special interest in the elderly, made a similar point (1973 : 47), yet one of the arguments frequently put to the Seebohm Committee was that the isolation of the home help service from the then children's department made it difficult for child care officers to utilise home helps in avoiding the need to receive children into residential care.

THE LOCAL AUTHORITY SYSTEM

To the client and his home help it may seem to be a matter of little importance whether the service is run by an elected local authority, an appointed public body, or is part of the civil service. Nevertheless, the overall framework within which the service operates and the way in which financial resources are allocated to it have profound effects on the quantity and quality of provision.

Local government is managed by elected representatives who are responsible to the electorate. Since the early 1970s, successive governments have sought to restrict the ability of local authorities to increase their expenditure, but within the totality of a local authority's budget the question of how much should be devoted to the development of the home help service is entirely a matter for elected representatives. They also have wide discretion as to how the service should be manned, the criteria adopted for allocating the service, and the training of home helps and organisers. Decisions that they make about the extent and quality of other services such as housing, old people's homes, social workers, occupational therapy services, and day centres also influence the way in which the home help service operates. The fact that local government is, as the words imply, *government locally*, means that systems, practices, procedures, priorities, and policies vary greatly from one area to another, making it difficult to generalise about how the service operates.

The Local Authority Social Services Act of 1970 and the Social Work (Scotland) Act of 1969, as amended by subsequent local government reorganisation, allocate social welfare functions, including responsibility for the home help service, to specific authorities. In England and Wales they are undertaken by non-metropolitan counties (39 in England, 8 in Wales), metropolitan districts (36), London boroughs (32), and the Common Council for the City of London. Scotland now provides home helps through its 9 regional councils. The law imposes certain constraints on the way in which local authorities exercise their social services powers. In England and Wales each social services authority must appoint a social services committee and only functions specified by law can be considered by that committee. In Scotland a similar provision applies. Each authority must appoint a director of social services (director of social work in Scotland), although, if desired, one director can be appointed to serve more than one authority.

Authorities with responsibilities for social services are also responsible for the education service in England (except inner London), Wales, and Scotland, but health services are administered separately by appointed authorities. In Northern Ireland social services and health provision are jointly managed by four boards, while education is the responsibility of separate boards.

In the metropolitan districts and London boroughs housing duties are administered by the authority that has social services functions, but in the counties and in Scotland housing is the responsibility of district councils. In Northern Ireland there is a separate housing executive covering the province. Nationally social services responsibilities are divided between the Secretary of State for Social Services in England and the Secretaries of State for Scotland, Wales, and Northern Ireland.

The overall pattern of services is confusing and reflects a series of compromises involving tradition, nods in the direction of devolution, and differing needs of urban and rural areas. The common factor throughout is that the home help service is regarded as an integral part of social welfare provision.

By any standard, local authorities are large organisations and are often the largest employer of labour within their areas. Their organisational structures follow a pattern similar to most other large organisations, with a chain of accountability that stretches from the shop floor to the top managers – in the case of local authorities, the elected representatives. Implicitly (and with certain minor exceptions) decisions by an employee of an authority are made on behalf of the council as a whole and the employee can, therefore, be asked to account for his actions. Even the behaviour of a home help in the home of a client can be debated by a full meeting of the council, although in practice problems, including many issues of policy, are settled by committees and sub-committees, while disputes or misunderstandings are ironed out by discussion and correspondence between elected members and senior staff.

In any organisation with two or more people, work is allocated by a system of delegation, each person being responsible for a segment of work or a range of duties. If the organisation is sufficiently large there will be further delegations within each work group. Thus, in a social services department the director of social services has delegated responsibility from the social services committee for the day-to-day work of the department, in accordance with any constraints laid down by the committee and the council in relation to policy, the provision of finance, and manpower. He, in turn, will allocate functions to other staff and hold them accountable for their performance. All domiciliary services may be grouped under an assistant director who will further delegate decisions to a variety of area staff, including specialist staff such as home help organisers. For their part, organisers delegate certain tasks to home helps. It is a complex system, much criticised and much misunderstood, but it does ensure that policies flow from democratically elected members who can be held accountable for the quality of provision and for expenditure. Without a chain of command no one would control the service.

As already indicated, social services departments are not the only services run by local authorities. Major services such as education, housing, highways, libraries, the fire service, and many others, are also included in their responsibilities. These services are placed under the responsibility of a committee either singly or in groups, so that an authority has perhaps five, six, or even more committees responsible for services, with chief officers responsible to them for the provision of services to the public. Without some central control these committees and the departments below them would be fighting one another for a bigger share of available resources, and it would be difficult to establish policies and priorities for the authority as a whole. To provide this central control and co-ordination, and to ensure that certain specialist advice and services are available to all committees and departments, most authorities have established a policy committee together with certain resource committees and departments to deal with finance, manpower, and property – the three key resources in the provision of any service. These committees and their matching departments establish procedures about the use of resources.

It can therefore be seen that although the social services committee and director of social services have delegated authority from the full council to decide certain policy issues relating to social services, their discretion to make decisions that affect the allocation of resources is severely limited. Usually the following types of decisions require the approval of a central resource department or committee.

Finance
(1) Increased expenditure.
(2) A switch of money from one budget heading to another.
(3) The write-off of a bad debt.

Property
(1) The acquisition or disposal of property.
(2) The repair, maintenance, or improvement of property and land.
(3) The change of use of property.

Manpower
(1) Recruitment arrangements.
(2) Variations to the staffing establishment.
(3) Variations to job descriptions.
(4) The grading and regrading of staff.
(5) The granting of special leave.
(6) Changes of policy which will involve consultation with trade unions.

In practice there is considerable discussion and interplay between staff in central resource departments and in departments providing services to the public, because all services are resource based. Very few changes of consequence can be effected by a social services committee or director of social services without reaching agreement with at least one and sometimes all three resource controllers.

In addition, certain other functions exercised in a social services department may be subject to control, consultation, or advice from another department. For example, legal matters will be handled by the council's solicitor and his staff; public relations and publicity, including the publication of leaflets and posters and the insertion of advertisements for recruitment, may be the responsibility of a centrally based press officer for the authority. Access to a computer is likely to be controlled from a central department; the provision of transport may be a function of the highways department and highways committee; fire prevention may be the responsibility of an officer in the fire brigade. There may be central officers dealing with research, safety, staff training, emergency services, energy conservation, and archives, as well as authority-wide arrangements for providing office accommodation, telephones, photo-copying, stationery, and advice on scientific matters such as the quality of foodstuffs and equipment.

During the past ten years local authorities have become very conscious of the need to adopt a corporate approach to their services and to maintain consistent policies throughout the council's activities. Inevitably this means that a new course of action requires the involvement of a large number of people from different departments, all of whom work to different sets of priorities, have different perceptions, and follow different timescales; they may also offer conflicting advice and may not have the delegated authority to commit their own department to an agreed course of action. Whilst a corporate approach brings certain advantages, no one will dispute that it can cause immense problems in a service like social welfare which must be constantly changing if it is to be effective. Many managers with key responsibilities feel that they do not control the services for which they are responsible, and at local level staff are often frustrated and bewildered by the delays that occur in reaching decisions, and the seemingly endless procedures required to obtain answers to matters of trivial importance.

Every year each local authority publishes a budget statement speci-fying, under numerous headings, the way in which it intends to spend its money the following year. The budget reveals the overt and covert policies of the authority. It indicates the balance of expenditure as between various services such as education, libraries, and social services; within social services it allocates finance between sections representing different client groups and between residential, day, and domiciliary provision.

Budget preparation is a complex operation that takes many months. During times when expenditure levels are rising, changes in policy can largely be accommodated by increased spending, but during a period of financial standstill or cutback increases in one area of activity may require reductions in another. Most local authority services make intensive use of labour which is an inflexible commodity. It is difficult to redeploy labour on new tasks. For example, in taking decisions to reduce the number of teachers or to cut library staff in order to transfer financial savings to improve home help provision, it cannot be assumed that the staff whose jobs are to be abolished will find their way into the home help service. There are immense problems for an authority wishing to reduce its labour force to save expenditure or to divert finance to another area of expenditure. Thus, local authorities tend to be slow-moving creatures that lumber towards distant goals, only to find that during the journey the goal posts have been moved.

Whilst the budget represents a snapshot of an authority's intentions and reveals the balance of expenditure afforded to different types of service, finance is not necessarily the key to change or to improving services. Whatever the total sum allotted it is possible to devise many different ways of allocating expenditure depending on the importance attributed to staff training, to the ratio of managers to home helps, and to a range of policy objectives. Once policies are determined, finance will regulate the extent of the service, but the quality will be a direct result of manpower policies – grading levels, organisation structures, job descriptions, recruitment policies, and industrial relations procedures.

In recent years local authorities have become increasingly conscious of the central role played by manpower policies in shaping services. A rapid reduction or redeployment of manpower presents so many problems that during times of financial uncertainty many authorities have arbitrarily frozen vacant posts; whilst this damages the service it usually saves expenditure and more importantly leaves the authority with greater flexibility to reorganise its services. The fewer people in post the easier it is to make changes: vacant posts do not object to change. In some authorities manpower budgets have become a more important constraint than finance; limitations placed on recruitment or on the overall number of staff in post can reduce services and expenditure just as effectively as direct financial cuts, but can do infinitely more harm to services if applied indiscriminately. Governments have sought to encourage a shift of employment from the public services to manufacturing industry and have urged local authorities to restrict the number of staff employed. By applying strict cash limits on grants to local authorities at a time of high inflation, governments have ensured that as salaries and wages rise, local authorities are under pressure to reduce staff numbers to keep costs within the specified overall limits.

Minimum standards are laid down in respect of some local authority services by central government, but there is considerable scope for variations between authorities. The allocation of resources between services within a local authority is a matter for political judgement. The various political parties and individuals within them differ in their views about the level of public expenditure that is justified and the extent to which different services should be developed. Whilst some elected members retain a global view of the affairs of their particular authority, probably the majority find it difficult to balance all the conflicting demands made upon resources and tend to support particular services with which they are familiar. If members of a social services committee wish to argue for more social services spending or seek to protect the service from cuts, it is necessary for them to marshal their arguments. The value of social services provision is not self-evident to everyone, particularly those who wish to see more money spent on protecting the environment, on improving education, maintaining transport and road systems, or building houses. Well-informed social services committee members, particularly those in the majority party, by arguing the case in private discussions, party meetings, and local authority committees, determine the share of resources allocated to social services.

DEPARTMENTAL STRUCTURE

There is a great diversity about the way in which local authorities arrange their internal structure to provide the home help service. The Department of Health and Social Security reported in 1973 that 'No two structures appear to be alike' (DHSS 1973 : 7) and this situation has not changed. The only common base for all services is that they are part of social welfare services and that decision-making about clients is decentralised. Beyond that there are no generalisations that apply.

Rowbottom, Hey, and Billis (1978 : 169) identified three basic models for the management of the home help service. These were, first, *outposting*, by which the service has its own hierarchical system, headed by a chief home help organiser based at headquarters with a management responsibility for the service and all who work in it; secondly, *attachment*, in which professional control is retained through a structure headed by a post in headquarters, whilst day-to-day operational control is in the hands of an area or district manager such as a principal social worker who has wider responsibilities; thirdly, there is *functional monitoring*, by which all control of the service is decentralised to area or district-based managers who have wider responsibilities, while headquarters staff retain a monitoring, advisory, and perhaps a planning role. The authors found that the latter two models were most common. This is not borne out by the London Boroughs Home Help Services Managers Group (1978 : 5) who found that in eighteen of the thirty-two London boroughs organisers were accountable to a centrally based officer. However, the findings of the National Council of Home Help Services (1979 : sect.2.4) confirm the views of Rowbottom *et al.*

The success of the home help service and its close involvement with the needs of the elderly have led many authorities to extend the duties of organisers to other services. The London Boroughs Home Help Services Managers Group (1978 : 42–6) found that many organisers administered additional services and also assessed needs on behalf of services administered by others. Out of thirty-two boroughs studied, assessments for the meals-on-wheels service were carried out by organisers in twenty-two, whilst in five others organisers were entirely responsible for the provision of meals-on-wheels services. In seven boroughs organisers provided a night-sitting service, in seven laundry services, and in six residential home care services. In one borough, organisers carried out assessments for laundry provision and in two they made assessments for day care.

The National Council of Home Help Services in 1979 received completed questionnaires from eighty-seven local authorities including the Scottish regions (but excluding Northern Ireland). It found field organisers heavily committed with neighbourly help (except in Scotland) with meals-on-wheels, night-sitting service, and to a lesser extent, laundry services.

The London Boroughs Home Help Services Managers Group (1978 : 43–4) found that home help provision was more likely to develop into an integrated caring service in those authorities where there was a central organiser with managerial responsibility for the service. The figures are quite startling – see *Table 3*.

Given the infinite variety of ways in which services can be structured and that organisations have developed piecemeal and haphazardly, it is important from time to time that managers examine the system currently operating in their authorities to determine whether it represents the most effective way of providing services. The key issue is whether there is an overwhelming need for the home help service to be a unified whole, with its own principal officer at headquarters with managerial responsibility for the service, and with organisers at area and district level working alongside but separate from other services such as social caseworkers, domiciliary and residential care. Powerful arguments can be advanced for this model, which is supported by home help organisers themselves and through their institute. The contrary view is put by some managers in related parts of social services departments who urge that the prime need

Table 3 *Table showing how the development of integrated home care services in London varies depending on whether or not there is a centrally based member of staff with overall responsibility for the service*

service integrated with home help service	boroughs with centrally based organiser		boroughs without centrally based organiser	
	number	%	number	%
meals-on-wheels	17	89	10	77
good neighbour	12	63	4	31
night-sitter	6	32	1	8
laundry	5	26	3	23
residential help	5	26	1	8
mobile unit	3	16	4	31
total boroughs	19	—	13	—

is for integrated domiciliary services at local level, and that this can only be achieved if all domiciliary services (and some would say day and residential services too) are accountable to one manager with direct responsibility for them all. We return to this matter in Chapter 11.

The London Boroughs Home Help Services Managers Group who researched services in London during 1976 were in no doubt about the need for a strong central direction of home help services. They felt that, without it, staff at local level interpreted and implemented policy in different ways resulting in 'varied practices, systems and delivery of service to clients'. The group felt that aspects 'such as co-ordination, monitoring, studying the service for future developments, effecting good systems, ensuring rationalisation of overall practice to provide efficient delivery to the client, warrants the full-time support of one centrally based management organiser' (1978 : 14).

Some authorities have created a post centrally within the social services department with full responsibility for developing home help services, but have placed the day-to-day management of the service with staff in the areas, leaving the centrally based member of staff with power to monitor, co-ordinate, and plan, but no ability to change the service. This style of management is not particularly successful. Indeed, advisers in social services departments who have no executive function are generally held in low regard. The Department of Health and Social Security, reviewing the position in 1973, stated:

'With so much variety in organisational structures it is hardly surprising that problems of dual accountability, co-ordination and supervision and occasionally of split administrative and operational arrangements can arise between social services department areas and headquarters and between different types and grades of staff. Many of these problems have still to be worked out.' (DHSS 1973 : 38)

Unlike the rest of the United Kingdom, in Northern Ireland the supervision of home helps is largely undertaken by social work assistants who carry out a variety of other duties. These duties vary from board to board, but include receiving applications for residential accommodation, specialised housing, meals-on-wheels, day care, and domiciliary laundry services. Social work assistants are responsible for assessing needs, recruiting home helps, and allocating the service. A research study found:

'The Assistants argued in favour of acting both as social workers for the elderly and as home help organisers for two reasons. First, their personal knowledge of the clients and the home helps facilitated mutually satisfactory placements. Secondly, their close contact with certain home helps could often reduce the need for them to visit since they could rely on the home helps to report any change in the client's condition.' (Stevenson 1977)

Although there are variations in the organisational pattern in different boards, each social work assistant generally forms part of a team of three or four who, together with three or four social workers, are responsible to a senior social worker who has responsibility for social work and home help services in his district. This model, supported by the Northern Ireland Central Personal Social Services Advisory Committee (1978 : 45), was endorsed by the Department of Health and Social Services in 1980 (Circular 1/80).

Organisational structures for the home help service differ so much between authorities that it is virtually impossible to present a readable and understandable summary. The fact that different authorities place different responsibilities on organisers, such as meals-on-wheels, night-sitters, and good neighbours schemes, makes it difficult to draw comparisons. Even authorities that appear on the surface to have adopted similar structures may allocate different duties to posts with similar titles, while posts that appear to carry the same responsibilities may have different titles and be placed on widely differing salary scales. The National Council of Home Help Services found that at least 11 different salary grades were used in Great Britain for organisers with direct responsibility for home helps (1979 : sect.2.6.3). Twelve grades were identified in respect of personnel who carried out authority-wide responsibilities for the home help service, but there was a considerable overlap between the grades of field organisers and principal organisers.

In the survey by the London Boroughs Home Help Services Managers Group (1978 : 6–9) it was found that for staff carrying authority-wide responsibility for home help services 11 different titles were used, and the salary grades ranged from AP4 to Principal Officer Scale 1 – which means that the highest grade was almost 50 per cent higher than the lowest.

The National Council of Home Help Services study (sect.2.6.3) also identified a number of authorities that employed an intermediate grade of management between field and principal organisers: 9 out of the 11 gradings identified in respect of these posts were identical to those of field organiser posts in other authorities. The same survey (sect.2.6.2) illustrates a variation of staff ratios so wide that it is simply not possible to offer any rational explanation, except to say that local people differ in their understanding and expectation of the service. Only such an explanation accounts for the fact that in Hertfordshire there were 30 home helps per organiser, whilst in Northumberland the ratio was 92, and in Gwent 96. In Inner London the ratio varied from 29 (Islington) to 54 (Wandsworth) and in Outer London from 24 (Hillingdon) to 50 (Waltham Forest). Who can explain why in Devon each organiser had an average 177 clients, and in Rotherham 179, while in Humberside and Mid-Glamorgan she had 575, and in Sandwell 627? The London Boroughs Home Help Services Managers Group (1978 : 13) found that the ratio of home helps to organising staff varied by a factor of 6 and that the ratio of clients per organiser varied by a factor of 7.

The Pearce working party reported that the ratios of organisers to full-time equivalent home helps ranged in England and Wales between 1 to 13 and 1 to 335 (Pearce Report 1974 : 10). The ratio recommended by the Institute of Home Help Organisers is 1 organiser to 25 home helps. Figures in Appendix 1 show that in 1980 the average number of cases per organiser in Wales was more than double that in Scotland, and that the ratio of cases per organiser averaged 179 in Scotland and 478 in Wales.

A small number of authorities have sought to reduce pressure on organisers by appointing assistant organisers and by creating the post of senior home help to share the workload. Such measures can only be regarded as reasonable if the staff concerned are adequately trained and experienced and properly remunerated for the responsibilities they carry. Trainee organisers are also sometimes used primarily to relieve hard-pressed organisers of routine work.

Considerable variations occur in the level of clerical support. Some tasks are variously carried out by organisers and clerks, by specialist staff in finance and personnel sections, or by staff in other departments; this makes direct comparison difficult. However, the ratio of clerical staff varies so much that it is impossible to explain differences in terms of different organisational patterns. The London Boroughs Home Help Services Managers Group (1978 : 32–3) collected information about the number of clerks attached to home help services. The ratio of clerks to clients ranges between 1 to 343 and 1 to 1,256. Hackney, with a caseload of 5,025 clients, employed 4 clerks – the same as Hillingdon, which had 1,899 clients. Lewisham, with a caseload of 4,948, had 11.5 clerks.

With such massive variations in the management of services it is barely possible to regard home help provision as a single service throughout Great Britain meeting similar needs. At best it is a diverse range of services attempting to meet a variety of human needs; at worst, it is a jumble of provision responding to the prejudices and whims of local pressure. Whatever else may be said, those managerially responsible for the service have not succeeded in providing it with a professional base.

Considering the number of staff employed on home help duties and the cost it is a matter of considerable surprise that the Department of Health and Social Security does not employ an experienced home help organiser to advise government ministers and local authorities about the development of services. One reason for this is that local authorities themselves provide too few opportunities for capable organisers to reach policy-making levels in social services departments; consequently, able and ambitious staff either do not join the service, or they move to posts where advancement is more readily available without becoming familiar with the authority-wide problems of running the home help service. It is perhaps significant that apart from small scale 'in house' studies, research into the home help service has been undertaken by staff from other disciplines.

5 · World-wide services

Although the home help service is often described as world-wide, it must be remembered that much of the world's population goes to bed hungry every night and faces death and disablement from diseases that have been largely conquered in western countries. Only when basic human needs for food, warmth, and shelter have been met and when medical care is generally available is it possible for a country to contemplate the development of State-supported home care services for the disadvantaged.

Forty-four organisations in seventeen countries were affiliated to the International Council of Home Help Services in 1982 – countries as diverse as Japan and Luxemburg, Finland, and Israel. In almost every case the service grew from a concern to reduce infant mortality by providing for mothers with young children and subsequently developed wider concerns until now the elderly represent the main clientele. Religious and voluntary organisations have played a prominent part in identifying needs and launching new services although, with a few exceptions, the State has assumed an increasingly important role in subsidising and supervising the provision. Germany is usually credited with having the first paid home help service – in Frankfurt in 1893 – a year ahead of England.

Few countries made much progress in developing services before the end of the second world war. Services started in France in 1920. Voluntary organisations were active in Sweden from 1920 when the Red Cross and other organisations were responsible for launching services modelled on those operating in England. The Red Cross also started the first Canadian Homemaker Service in Toronto in the 1920s. Belgium, Holland, Norway, and Finland could all boast modest services provided by voluntary organisations before the outbreak of the second world war. In Finland a voluntary child welfare organisation started the service in 1930, and by 1939 it had developed a five-month training course: those who passed the examinations were entitled to a badge and a uniform. Services in Germany which developed strongly after 1925 were dissolved by the Nazi government in 1933 and did not recommence until 1945. A formalised service was established in the United States stimulated largely by a conference in Washington in 1939. By 1958 over 100 agencies were providing a homemaker service in the United States, mainly for families with young children; provision was concentrated in the east and in large cities, while seventeen states had no service.

As in the United Kingdom, the end of the second world war marked a new beginning for social welfare services throughout the western world. The hardships of war broke down social barriers; there was a prevailing wish, not merely to rebuild war-torn cities, but to reconstruct society in a way that would protect the vulnerable, promote social justice, and enhance the dignity of the individual. Social welfare services underwent rapid change and would have expanded overnight had the necessary resources been available.

In 1947 the Belgian and Norwegian governments began subsidising home help services. Legislation brought into force in 1949 made Denmark's municipalities responsible for services that had been begun by voluntary initiative. Similar legislation had been introduced in Sweden in 1944. Services in the Netherlands, although subsidised by the State, were provided mainly by religious organisations: the Protestant Church operated in the north of the country and the Roman Catholic Church in the south. A third voluntary organisation – the Humanistic – offered help to people of no denomination. At this time services in New Zealand and Australia were administered by voluntary committees subsidised by the State.

By 1952 France had services provided by voluntary organisations and private initiative which received State subsidies; the service was available throughout France and extended to North African colonies. At this time provision in Canada, Austria, Italy, and the United States was operated without public subsidy. In Helsinki, Finland, a local authority home help service was launched in 1951. At first it was available only to families with children, but following new regulations in 1967 it was extended to include the elderly and handicapped; now the elderly absorb about 70 per cent of the service.

Services in Switzerland began in about 1950 by voluntary initiative and provision was later developed by local authorities. The service in Israel was founded in 1958 in Tel Aviv. After an initial success it was extended to Haifa in 1961 and then Jerusalem; special services were later provided for families containing mental illness and mental handicap. Japan's service commenced during 1956 in the Nagano prefecture. In 1960 the Japanese Ministry of Labour began a campaign to promote the home help service within industry; the objective set out by the ministry included 'First, improving the welfare of workers' families, secondly, developing new occupations of women and modernising domestic work' (Mayumi 1962 : 5). Within two years the ministry reported that 70 schemes were in operation and that 250 women had undertaken a special four-week training course for home helps.

By the early 1970s countries as diverse as Iceland, Spain, Barbados, and Hong Kong were developing home help services. There were and are great similarities between services in different countries, but it is difficult to make direct comparisons. The type and level of social security payments, the organisation of health care, and the nature of social welfare provision vary enormously, as does the kind of structure through which services are provided. A general feature reported by most countries is that domestic help is poorly paid and has a low status. As a preparation for the International Congress of Home Help Services held in Stockholm in May 1981, Kerstell and Unge, from the National Swedish Board of Health and Welfare, visited Switzerland, France, Belgium, and the Netherlands. They found that despite developments in training, the home help service continued to be a low-paid occupation, almost entirely restricted to women, carrying little status, and tending to represent a transitory occupation accepted 'for lack of other or better ones' (1981 : 7). Similar observations have been made about the position in Japan although special attempts were made in the early days to entice into the service 'women of middle age who have stayed at home for a long time, doing domestic work and taking care of children' (Mayumi 1962 : 6). Even in countries with high levels of unemployment it is sometimes difficult to recruit to the service. To combat the problems of low status and increased demand, many countries have invested heavily in training schemes and in the development of special services to meet particular social needs.

Staff training has played an important part in nearly every service. A training programme of one to two years is common. The United Kingdom appears to be almost alone in leaving the training of home helps to *ad hoc* local arrangements. In the early 1950s the Austrian family help service established training courses extending over six months. In France at that time training included cookery, dietetics, practical housekeeping, budgeting, dressmaking, mending, laundry, hygiene, and the care of children. At an international conference held in London in 1952 a French delegate said that trained home helps received a diploma and that the work was looked upon in France as a profession. At the same conference emphasis was laid on training by delegates from Belgium, Holland, Sweden, and Norway; Finland had an intensive training scheme for home helps lasting two years as long ago as 1945.

The gap between the United Kingdom and most other countries in the provision of training for home helps has widened in recent years. In 1970 in the Netherlands home help training was undertaken in twenty-four training schools providing courses lasting eighteen months, with subjects including domestic science, child care, social work, psychology, and religious training. All the 26,500 home helps employed in the Netherlands in 1970 were qualified. By the same year Switzerland had nine training schemes providing an eighteen-month training in housekeeping, cooking, dietetics, babycare, care of the elderly, anatomy, first aid, social sciences, law, and psychology; this training was followed by nine months' work under supervision in nursing homes, hospitals, and with families. In Germany twenty-one training schools provide a one-year theoretical training followed by a second year of practical training in the field. Because of recruitment problems a new home help training school was opened in Helsinki in 1980.

Some countries have found it expedient to develop a two-tier system so that home helps undertaking rehabilitative work, and those whose work content includes special caring functions, receive more elaborate training. In Belgium a one-year training course has been developed for home helps who wish to work with families, whilst those who work with the elderly follow a five-month course. Attempts to integrate domiciliary services for the elderly in Sweden have led to the development of advanced training for young people who, it is hoped, will make a career in the home help service. A special grade of homemakers are employed in Sweden to undertake rehabilitative work with multi-problem families; they receive a more advanced training and have higher rates of pay. Finland has homemakers who are trained to help families with children and home helpers who care mainly for the elderly and the handicapped; in exceptional circumstances home helps feed pets and tend farm animals, but many Finnish local authorities run a separate relief service for farmers with animals in the event of illness. The Netherlands differentiates in the training and deployment of home helps who work with families as opposed to the elderly; it also provides a special service for multi-problem families, utilising specially trained home helps.

The Jerusalem homemaker service has developed provision to meet the needs of families with mentally handicapped children; under the supervision of occupational therapists, specially trained homemakers meet the personal care needs of the child and assist him or her to develop maximum physical skills by structured play and physical exercises.

In Chicago, Illinois, two categories of service were developed by a voluntary organisation as part of a project to assist the aged. They included housekeeping for the client whose primary need was for assistance with household chores, and the homemaker service where 'the interest and personal warmth that the homemaker brought into the relationship had a lot to do with the elderly person's improved self-concept and interest in obtaining health care and other needed services' (Davis 1977 : 5).

In Germany and Switzerland there are strong nursing components in training schemes reflecting the personal caring role and nursing activities of the service in those countries. About 30 per cent of Japanese home helps have a licence to nurse. Some medical insurance companies in Germany and the United States include payment for home help service within their range of benefits. In countries where private medical insurance plays a significant part in meeting the costs of health care, it is sometimes reported that since the home help service is not similarly covered there is an incentive for patients to remain in hospital longer than is strictly necessary. In the United States home help services are provided by private and voluntary organisations, often under contract to health and social welfare services; this led to a remark by one leading organiser at a recent international conference, that the first essential of a home help service in the United States was the employment of a good accountant.

The Constitution of the International Council of Home Help Services (1981) provides a definition of home help services which emphasises the origin of the need that is met rather than the objectives of the service or a description of the tasks performed. The definition signifies that home help work 'is given by qualified persons under competent direction, generally for a limited period of time in order to assist the family unit or individual in cases of illness, overwork, incapacity, absence of one of the parents, maternity, old age and other social or health reasons'.

Problems of definition make it difficult to assemble reliable comparative data about the extent of home help provision in different countries. Even within countries there are differences in the way in which similar work is recorded. Night-sitters may be variously regarded as part of the home help service or as a separate provision depending on the way they are organised and deployed. Similarly, duties in relation to home bathing may be an integral part of home help provision or an aspect of duties undertaken by auxiliaries in home nursing services. In most countries a significant proportion of home helps are engaged on a part-time basis, and published figures seldom reveal the average number of hours worked by employees.

It is important to bear in mind these shortcomings when considering statistical information about the service. However, within these limitations the following table, compiled by Mikio Mori in 1973 and reproduced from his book in Japanese, *Home Help*, is an indication of the extent of services in sixteen countries at that time.

Table 4   *Home help provision 1973*

name of country	number of home helps	ratio/100,000 population
Sweden	65,700	825
Norway	22,231	577
Netherlands	52,130	405
Great Britain	67,439	138
Finland	4,556	97
Belgium	4,018	42
Switzerland	2,060	33
Canada	5,000	23
West Germany	11,203	19
United States	30,000	15
France	7,144	14
Japan	9,220	9
Israel	273	9
Austria	355	5
Australia	30	0.2
Italy	50	0.1

Mori's study was by no means complete. It does not include Denmark, where it was reported in 1971 that 100,000 home helps were employed, or Iceland, where 35 staff were employed in Reykjavik. It seems likely that in 1973 upwards of 300,000 home helps were employed world-wide.

Since 1973 many countries have reported significant developments. By 1980 the number of home helps in the United States was said to have increased from 30,000 to 100,000, the number in Switzerland and Great Britain had risen by more than 50 per cent, and a further 12,800 were employed in Sweden. It seems likely that the figure of 400,000 home helps in member countries of the International Council of Home Help Services, quoted by Kemm in 1977 (p.106), was an accurate estimate, and it is probably realistic to assume that approximately 500,000 home helps are now employed in western countries and Japan. About one in five is employed full time.

As provision developed national organisations were created to bring together those responsible for directing and managing services. The International Council of Home Help Services was inaugurated in 1959. Membership consisted of national agencies in Belgium, Austria, Denmark, Finland, France, Germany, Israel, Italy, the Netherlands, Norway, Sweden, Switzerland, the United Kingdom, and the United States. Denmark and Italy discontinued membership but Japan and Australia subsequently joined; Canada, Iceland, and Luxemburg became full members in 1980. Regular international conferences and seminars have been held drawing together staff from voluntary organisations, local authorities, and central government, together with political representatives from many diverse countries. These have proved invaluable opportunities to explore common problems concerned with organisational issues and service delivery.

Since the mid-1970s a succession of speakers from many different countries at international conferences on the home help service have emphasised the impact of economic recession on plans for developing services. Andersen, representing the Local Government Research Institute on Public Administration and Finance in Denmark, suggested at the Stockholm international congress in 1981 that staff in health and social services were apprehensive about the future because,

> 'after a number of years of expansion and of general public understanding, many now tend to believe that we will face a decade of stagnation, maybe even recession; years with brutal fight between social groups, each of which will try to conquer a bigger share of a diminishing cake with the inevitable result that the weaker groups – the aged, the sick and the unorganised – will lose.'   (1981 : 1)

He felt, however, that there was room for optimism in so far as a shortage of funds would stimulate better systems of organisation and lead to greater experimentation in the provision of services.

Dr P. Gilliand, Lecturer for Social Policy at the University of Geneva, echoed the views of many when he told the Montreux international congress in 1977: 'The collective consciousness of the limits of resources is now developing which demands in the first place a struggle against waste and a reorganisation of the social services. Economic growth, as necessary as it may be, favours the quantitative aspects often to the detriment of the qualitative ones' (1977 : 87). On the other hand, Mats Hulth from the Stockholm municipality in Sweden told the Stockholm conference:

> 'All Swedish district authorities are now being forced to try to save money in as many areas as possible and in many cases this may bring

about cuts and savings in the home help services too. Each home help may be allocated more pensioners to help in the same amount of time as before, and the pensioners themselves may be subjected to a more rigorous needs test and obtain help more seldom than before.'

SPECIAL SCHEMES

Social and health vehicle in Finland (Kivela 1981)

As in other western countries Finland's elderly population has been increasing. In rural areas houses often lack basic amenities and there is a tendency for the elderly to live in the poorest accommodation. A study in 1976 found that 12 per cent of persons over the age of 74 had no electricity supply and that 76 per cent had outside toilets, whilst about 45 per cent of this age group needed assistance in cooking, cleaning, washing clothes, and shopping.

Responsibility for the care of the elderly in Finland is divided between health and social welfare services. Much thought has been given to ways of improving co-operation between all the staff concerned, particularly those working in domiciliary services. Research evidence in 1978 suggested that there was no lack of willingness to co-operate but that new administrative arrangements were required to ensure close working relationships.

Since 1971 the home help service in Finland has been operating home service cars equipped with radio telephones and carrying cleaning materials including vacuum cleaners. By 1977, twenty-seven communes were deploying such vehicles. Under the Finnish Public Health Act of 1972 health services were also permitted to equip and operate mobile units, and an experimental clinic car was introduced into the commune of Kuusano in 1978, enabling a nurse with sophisticated equipment to visit and advise the elderly.

In the following year a combined social and health service vehicle was provided on an experimental basis in the commune of Posio. Apart from providing a viable service for the elderly, it was hoped that this provision would help to secure closer working relationships between the home care service and home nurses. Posio is a rural area in the north of Finland with a total population of 6,115, having a lower proportion of elderly persons than in the country as a whole, 8.5 per cent being over the age of 64 years. The vehicle is described as a delivery truck and contains a washing machine, sewing machine, iron, vacuum cleaner, and other cleaning equipment and cleaning materials. For medical and nursing care it contains a medicine chest, a blood pressure gauge, stethoscope, otoscope, air injector, thermometer, wheelchair, stretcher, electro-cardiogram, haemoglobinometer, and other apparatus.

To help meet the personal care needs of infirm and isolated old people, the vehicle carries a shower basin, brushes, combs, nail clippers, scissors, and razors. Laundry baskets, water carriers, and a refrigerator are also provided. As a stark reminder of the harshness of the elements and the bleakness of the terrain in the Arctic Circle the vehicle carries an electric generator, assorted tools such as a hammer, saw, and axe, together with a spade – the latter being an essential item of equipment of home help services in northern climes. To complete the equipment the vehicle has supplies of food, a coffee maker, and heavy-duty clothing for staff.

The vehicle is staffed by two home assistants (home helps) employed by the social welfare services and a nurse who is on the staff of the health services, thus ensuring close collaboration of the two organisations concerned with the domiciliary care of the elderly. The home assistants undertake the full range of tasks normally carried out by home helps, including chopping and carrying wood, carrying water, and baking. They also carry out personal care functions such as haircutting, shaving, and attending to feet. A particularly unusual feature is that the home assistants supply magazines and loan books. The home nurses share some of these tasks but also undertake the range of tasks associated with health visiting, home and clinic nursing. Staff in the vehicle liaise with the relatives of clients, neighbours, and voluntary organisations, in order to mobilise all available resources to support the elderly.

Some recent developments in Sweden

Services in Sweden have developed rapidly in recent years with many innovative schemes. The isolation of home helps causes particular problems, for they work alone and have few opportunities for contact with their organiser or with one another. In Stockholm over 110 domestic help bureaux have been established where home helps can meet their organisers and colleagues. The bureaux have facilities for preparing and eating meals and for taking a shower. Staff training sessions are held on the premises and special items of equipment are available. The bureaux are also used as centres for the distribution of frozen food to clients; this has been found to be more economical than home helps preparing meals.

Forty per cent of the work in Stockholm is undertaken in the homes of the elderly. Approximately 5 per cent of home helps are male; although some pensioners object to male home helps, saying a man cannot do the job, others have specifically requested a male help 'because they found them more fun' (Stockholm Social Welfare Board 1981 : 7).

In order to ensure the rapid availability of the service when bureaux are closed at weekends and after hours, an emergency telephone number is available to pensioners in Stockholm; during 1980, 104,000 calls were made to and from this number. The emergency telephone also carries text telephones for deaf persons. Some deaf home helps have been appointed who use sign language and this aids communication with deaf clients.

In 1980 Stockholm also introduced domestic help buses to facilitate the transport of home helps and cleaning equipment. As an experiment they have been fitted with radio communication. Teams of six home helps provided with a bus equipped with machines and utensils visit homes and carry out a thorough spring clean as necessary; the team will clean cupboards and wardrobes and send clothes to the laundry and dry cleaners. Several buses have been used in remote areas of Sweden; they carry food and other items, provide laundry facilities, and supply magazines and books.

In the far north of Sweden experimental schemes have been developed involving home helps in sheltered housing schemes for the younger physically handicapped. Home helps work closely with handicapped tenants, assisting them with a range of personal and domestic chores. Explaining why home helps are preferred to other personnel, the National Board of Health and Welfare says 'good home helpers, i.e. those with initiative and interest in the work, with their practical experience of ordinary everyday life, make excellent educationalists' (1981 : 7). As a result of the initial experiment it has been decided that home helps allocated to sheltered housing schemes will also continue some duties to the severely handicapped in their own homes. It is thought that this will prevent home helps becoming institutionalised and, at the same time, enable sheltered housing schemes to serve as training centres for a larger number of staff.

Sweden is a large but sparsely populated country. Trelleborg in the south is as near to Naples as it is to the northern boundary. Because of the distances involved, rural postmen serve as mobile post offices as well as delivering mail. Since 1974 the Swedish Post Office has offered social services authorities the opportunity of purchasing a number of additional services through rural postmen including regular contact with pensioners and the delivery of goods. Currently 2,600 rural postmen daily serve one million people (Swedish Post Office 1981).

Home help services and psychiatric care in the United States

The development of new drug treatments in the mid-1950s revolution-ised psychiatric care in the western world. Not only were periods of in-patient care shortened but patients who had been in hospital for many years were discharged in large numbers. In some countries the number of patients in psychiatric beds has fallen by 50 per cent during the past thirty years. Many schemes have been devised and operated linking home helps with specialist staff to offer support and care for discharged psychiatric patients. Details of a number of schemes were assembled by the National HomeCaring Council, formerly the National Council for Homemaker–Home Health Aide Service, USA, for the 1981 International Congress of Home Help Services in Stockholm, and we summarise here a description of these schemes.

The Indiana State Hospital at Evansville undertook a three-year demonstration project to ascertain the value of homemaker services in a psychiatric treatment programme. The service could be provided prior to admission, during treatment, or following discharge from hospital. The object of the service was to minimise the feeling of loss and trauma for the patient and his family, to prevent admission or readmission to hospital, to shorten hospital stay where admission became necessary, and to maintain the co-operation of the patient and his family throughout treatment. The homemaker also provided the hospital team with information about home conditions. The project is said to have proved satisfactory in achieving its objective.

The New York State Psychiatric Institute has developed a programme employing family aides recruited from the inner-city community surrounding the hospital to work with the patient and his family by reducing stress and preventing hospital admission. As in the Evansville project it was found that para-professionals not only provided direct benefits to the families concerned but supplied information and insights not otherwise available to the hospital team. At the end of the experimental project the family aides were absorbed on the payroll of the State hospital.

A demonstration and research project was developed in Baltimore by the Maryland Department of Mental Hygiene together with the Family and Children's Society. The project was concerned to identify what help was required to enable mothers to participate in community treatment and enhance their own role as mothers and housewives. A careful study of the outcome showed that homemakers could pose a considerable threat to the role of a wife and mother who was struggling to maintain her position within the family. With other families the initial reaction to the homemaker service was a rapid withdrawal from domestic and parental responsibilities; whilst this was seen as a therapeutic process, further help was required to re-educate the parents to resume their caring roles. During the two-and-a-half years of the demonstration project it was estimated that homemakers prevented the need for thirty-nine mentally ill parents to enter hospital. Ninety per cent of the mentally ill parents concerned were thought to have benefited from the work of the treatment team, made up of psychiatrist, social worker, and homemaker. The detailed involvement and responsibility of the treatment team in the care of the children made it necessary to abandon conventional methods of service delivery so that help could be provided at any time of the day or night if a crisis occurred.

A demonstration project in Ohio by the Cleveland Homemaker Service had features similar to the Baltimore project. Its aim was 'to sustain the family as a unit during the crisis of the mother's illness and to restore her to optimal level of functioning in her home as wife and mother'. It was commonly found that the mothers were withdrawn and indifferent to the maternal role. The service tended to concentrate on home management and child care tasks which required the least co-operation from the mother. Objectives with the highest frequency of failure were those involving teaching and encouraging.

A programme devised in North Essex, Massachusetts, between a community mental health centre and homemaker agency employed a consultant psychiatric nurse as the linchpin of the joint effort. A number of social agencies refer clients to the programme. The psychiatric nurse, in consultation with the referring agency, makes an assessment of the need. As in other projects already described, the homemaker has a unique opportunity to monitor the patient's mental state and to keep relevant professionals informed of changes as they occur. In some cases the personal relationship forged between the homemaker and the patient enables her to encourage the patient to seek further treatment. A significant finding arising from the project has been that with the passage of time and the development of greater expertise homemakers have become more skilful at detecting changes in the patient and communicating those changes to the psychiatric team.

The United States National HomeCaring Council has identified some of the key issues surrounding these special schemes. Perhaps the most obvious and therefore most likely to be overlooked is that although psychiatric services have been dominated by professional staff there is a clear and distinct role for para-professional staff working as part of a team. They can help prevent serious breakdown and enable patients to make a smooth transition from hospital to normal life in the community. They can also contribute to the understanding of the therapeutic team. Basic training suggested for all homemaker home health aides in the United States is a minimum of sixty hours. Training programmes orientated for homemakers serving the psychiatrically ill varied from a few hours to ninety-six hours spread over an eight-week period; mostly the training programmes lasted two or three weeks and were followed by continuing in-service training.

The need for professional supervision and support to enable home-makers to respond adequately to complex and sometimes threatening situations was apparent in all the schemes. In particular it was found necessary to provide opportunities for the homemaker to discuss problems that were stressful to her. Continuity between homemaker and professional supervisor appeared to be important. It was found that homemakers from the same cultural and economic background as the person served were able to develop a rapport more quickly. Staff perceived as non 'mental health' were seen by patients as providing home management and practical assistance rather than treatment and were therefore sometimes more easily accepted.

Agencies commonly found that homemakers were unable to serve at peak efficiency if they regularly worked an eight-hour day with the mentally ill; they performed better if they had a mixed workload including cases offering less demanding and more immediately gratifying situations. Improved staff morale and a higher quality of service were thought to follow from a full recognition of the skills and abilities of homemakers. Continuing education and experience with families under stress and a growing recognition by the therapeutic team should, it was felt, be recognised by advancement in the agency. Successful recruitment was seen as depending on the status afforded to the position of homemaker and the provision of incentives.

Intensified family help – an experiment in Finland (Majuri 1981)

An experiment was started in eight Finnish localities in 1976 to provide a specialist home help service for multi-problem families. At the core of the scheme was the homemaker, a senior grade of home help. Her dual function was to maintain standards of care and cleanliness and to guide the family, with special emphasis on helping its members to function more appropriately.

In order to ensure that the experimental scheme could be properly tested under normal working conditions, no additional staff or other resources were provided. The purpose of the project was:

(1) to broaden the scope of the homemaker's work and raise the prestige of the profession;
(2) to promote co-operation between different branches of social welfare, health care, and training, and to learn how to facilitate this co-operation;

(3) to discover when and under what conditions intensified family help would produce results;

(4) to study working methods.

Homemakers, and in most cases their immediate superiors (known as leading homemakers), attended special training courses for between one and two weeks. Each family was assigned a project supervisor drawn from an agency which had a particular interest in that family. Project supervisors were mainly psychologists and social workers from child guidance clinics, health centres, mental health clinics, and social welfare offices. Regular meetings were arranged between the homemaker and the project supervisor to discuss progress and to ensure that professional advice was made available. A special feature of the scheme was that the project supervisor was not merely a consultant; he or she remained responsible for the work undertaken and had a continuing involvement with the family.

At the outset a plan was drawn up for each family specifying the particular objectives of the service and the targets that were to be met. As far as possible members of each family were involved in discussions about the service, its content and purpose. Full notes were made by home-makers on each visit describing what took place. These notes formed the basis for regular discussions with project supervisors. Reports from homemakers and project supervisors were supplied to a central point for analysis.

In most cases the homemaker concentrated on domestic activities during the initial settling-in period; then the emphasis slowly changed so that the homemaker was performing an educative role, helping the family to organise itself more effectively and encouraging parents to develop their own abilities. The homemaker was not expected to provide specialist services. Her task was to encourage clients to seek assistance from experts. Examples of the work undertaken are:

(1) showing parents better methods of child care and upbringing;
(2) persuading parents that a child needed some kind of specialist assistance – for example, speech therapy – and helping them to get it;
(3) encouraging parents with drink or mental health problems to seek specialist help;
(4) working to improve relationships between family members;
(5) encouraging family members to seek outside contacts, relating perhaps to training, jobs, and leisure pursuits.

Homemakers worked with families for periods ranging from a few weeks to two years and generally reduced the frequency of visits with the passage of time. Sixty-five families with 170 children were assisted during the course of the five-year life of the project. A range of social problems was involved including unemployment, sickness, mental health problems, drink problems, low standards of housekeeping, emotional problems of children, poor family relationships, and difficult relationships with other people and with public authorities.

The project organisers are cautious about claiming too much for the impact of the service on the families concerned, particularly as it is difficult to assess the extent to which any improvement in family functioning will be permanent. However, they have noted improvements in parents' attitudes towards their children, including an increased understanding of how to relate to them and show affection. Many of the mothers were thought to have gained in confidence and to have achieved higher standards of housekeeping. The project organisers noted the danger of a housewife already lacking in self-assurance being further discouraged by observing an efficient and competent homemaker at work. Children's emotional disturbances and their symptoms were said to be relieved, including bedwetting and school phobia. Some children were brought to the attention of child guidance clinics, speech therapists, or day centres. In several instances an alcoholic father was persuaded to seek treatment.

Some families could not be helped – particularly those with multi-problems of long duration. However, even where no clear results could be demonstrated there are thought to have been improvements in the sense of security of the children. The best success was achieved in families confronted by a sudden crisis. Young families, whose difficulties had more recently arisen, were most willing to accept help, and the organisers suspect that early intervention by an intensive service prevented the development of more serious problems.

The project succeeded in demonstrating the flexibility of the homemaker's skills and enhanced her reputation with other professionals. The specialist guidance of the project supervisors was felt to be a particularly useful means of extending the value of the homemaker. The fact that the project brought together a number of different professionals helped to develop co-operation between various groups of staff in health and welfare services.

The homemakers themselves sometimes found the experience of working with such families very stressful and made good use of the expert guidance available. It was thought that in any long-term project it would be necessary to ensure that individual homemakers had a break from their work from time to time, perhaps returning to ordinary home help work for a period, in order to reduce stress.

When the experiment ended a number of local authorities in Finland incorporated this method of working in their service. An intensive family service began in Helsinki in 1979 for multi-problem families; a support group of social workers is available in respect of each family. In order to maximise the potential of homemakers, basic and supplementary training is being increased with special reference to the educative role homemakers can play with families. The success of the project has encouraged the Finnish National Boards of Social Welfare and Health to launch a joint experimental project to assist handicapped persons and to make them more independent.

6 · Objectives and policies

Numerous attempts have been made to state the objectives of home help services, but most of these endeavours have led to statements of such a general nature that they have little practical value in terms of setting targets for the service or enabling an assessment to be made of the extent to which performance matches those targets. A general statement of objectives might be:

> To provide skilled personnel who are flexible in their approach to the different conditions under which clients live, sensitive to clients' disabilities and needs, and aware of the range and purpose of other services provided.

Such a statement, however, tells us nothing about how priorities are to be determined or the nature and extent of the service.

This is a familiar problem in the social sciences; it is often difficult for medical officers, teachers, social workers, and many other groups of staff in the caring professions to be precise about their objectives, and they are beset by doubts – or they should be – about whether they are satisfactorily meeting the demands made upon them. Nevertheless, unless attempts are made to specify the purpose of services, the clients that can best be helped, and the skills required, instead of one home help service there will be as many different types of service as there are people employed in it.

It is a distinguishing mark of professional activity that its practitioners endeavour to evaluate their service and their skills, so that a distinctive body of knowledge is assembled which is refined by experiment and practice and which enables those concerned to share common goals. Despite the considerable growth in home help provision, knowledge about how decisions are made regarding the allocation of the service and on what basis is very sketchy. It is largely for this reason that the growth of the service in terms of expenditure and the number of clients helped has not been matched by a growth in status for those employed in it; from being an ancillary service to nurses and midwives in public health departments, the home help service has become ancillary to social work. With proper leadership, training, and recognition the service can and should become a profession in its own right with organisers working alongside other professionals, bringing their own distinctive skills to bear on human problems. Only when organisers are seen to exercise professional judgements based on a common body of knowledge, and when they can demonstrate that they have distinctive skills, equal but different to those of health visitors, home nurses, and social workers, will the service begin to achieve its full potential.

One of the key differences between home help organisers and other professional groups in the caring professions is that the organiser largely achieves her professional purpose through the control and direction of other paid staff. As well as having the necessary skill and knowledge to assess the needs of individual clients and their families, she must possess the administrative, financial, and management talents necessary to deploy a substantial workforce in a productive and economical way.

Good management revolves around objectives – how they are set and the resources in terms of manpower and equipment that are needed to achieve them. Organisations are established to achieve desirable objectives, and unless all those involved have a clear idea of what they are there will be muddle, confusion, and wasted effort. The home help service must learn from the mistakes of the social work profession. In the post-Seebohm era it was confidently expected that extensive social work services would solve many social problems, but the role of social workers was not defined. There was no consensus about their purpose, the extent to which they should defend clients against public policies or help them acquiesce. As a consequence there developed bitterness, frustration, and conflict among staff. The militancy and unrest that has characterised relations between social workers and their employers in some local authorities has not arisen because social workers have higher principles than other staff, or because their values differ from the managers who supervise them, but because the purpose of social work is too vague, and because the objectives being pursued are so fragmented and obscure that even when they are achieved there is no evidence to show the outside world that social work intervention has played a part. While the social work profession has valiantly sought to serve its clients and employing authorities, the uncertainty surrounding the nature of the social work task has created a restless anxiety, an apprehension and a discontent that can erupt like a volcano against employers when honest differences of view prevail between social workers and others.

But setting clear objectives is only the beginning. Unless objectives are achievable there will be staff unrest and services will not be cost effective or realise their full potential. Organisers at local level need to feel that they can meet the expectations of senior management for their geographical area, and home helps must feel that they can achieve the tasks set by their organiser. A small disparity between objectives and performance can stimulate constructive discussion and an analysis of the changes which may be required to bring targets and achievement into closer alignment. However, a significant gap between what is desired and what is achieved serves only to raise tension and anxiety among the workforce.

It is the task of management to set realistic objectives and to ensure that the means for achieving them are provided. In the absence of sufficient resources, objectives must be redefined otherwise there will be discord and dissatisfaction at all levels in the service. One of the key resources of a caring service is the expertise of staff. Managers must ensure not only that staff with appropriate experience and skills are appointed, but also that staff training schemes raise the quality of work so that skilled staff are available in sufficient numbers to meet the objectives of the service. Public services cannot begin to meet all the demands made upon them. The art of successful management is to keep objectives and resources in balance so that whatever the pressure placed upon the service by members of the public, staff are clear about their response.

THE CONTEXT

The home help service is part of a network of caring services, each of which has a role to play in supporting dependent people in the community. The extent and quality of care provided by public agencies in a given locality are determined not merely by the level of public expenditure or even the skills deployed, but by the extent to which those responsible for the management of services perceive themselves as providing an integrated caring service.

It is impossible to plan the provision of a home help service without making assumptions about the role of home nurses, health visitors, occupational therapists, social workers, and voluntary organisations. If these assumptions are wide of the mark the service will squander its resources. Managers at all levels need to be in constant communication with staff in other services to ensure that there is the fullest mutual understanding of policies and procedures. Services must be planned and operated jointly so that the impact of new policies is understood by all concerned. For example, the development of sheltered housing units by a housing authority, the extension of a geriatric day hospital, or the opening of an assessment unit for the physically handicapped may all have a profound effect on the operation of home help services. Planning for new services too often proceeds without reference to the impact of change elsewhere within the caring system.

However well developed the service becomes it can never, in isolation, provide effective care for an individual in need; it must be part of a wider package of care, one aspect of a network of caring services seeking to meet total needs. In many instances the clients' own families are the main carers, but for the client who lives alone with no relatives or friends at hand it is important that the organiser communicates with the general practitioner, health visitor, or home nurse who, depending on the circumstances, will have responsibility for some aspects of the client's well-being. The organiser will need to seek advice from other relevant professionals who know the client and inform them of any significant changes in the client or in the provision of service that may affect their contribution to the care provided.

If good relationships are forged the service can add to the knowledge of other professionals and assist them greatly in determining future treatment and patterns of care. In many instances the home help is in a better position than any other person to know how the client lives his life and to assess his capacity for self-care. As the Harvard Davis Report on group practice stated, 'The home help is a valuable source of information about changes in the patient's condition' (1971 : 37). This is confirmed by a number of studies including some in the United States. It is important that channels of communication between all the caring professions at forward planning and day-to-day operational levels are kept open.

By their nature, professional groups tend to be isolated from one another; they are quick to accuse and often display an abysmal ignorance of the way in which parallel professions operate. Each profession tends to see its own function as central to the care of clients with others performing subsidiary roles. Unless all professionals come together to define their respective responsibilities, omissions and overlaps will occur, causing clients to suffer and leading to a waste of scarce resources. In a study of hospital discharge arrangements for the elderly, Geraldine Amos interviewed general practitioners, health visitors, social workers, hospital doctors, and ward sisters. She concluded that many saw themselves as key to the provision of services, but that none accepted responsibility for seeing that all the necessary services for discharged elderly patients were provided (Amos 1975 : 20).

A study team from the Department of Health and Social Security which examined statistical and research evidence expressed the view that there was an overlap of function between home nurses and home helps in England (DHSS 1981b : 49). Nursing auxiliaries in particular were found to be performing some functions that were indistinguishable from those performed by home helps. In so far as this situation has developed on a casual or unintended basis, it is a reflection on the extent to which there is a lack of understanding between health and social services authorities. However, it must be recognised that in the late 1970s central government policy favoured a modest growth in health service expenditure and a considerable reduction for the personal social services; in addition, there was extreme pressure on local authorities to reduce their manpower requirements. A white paper published in November 1979 setting out government plans for Great Britain, *The Government's Expenditure Plans 1980–81*, suggested that the National Health Service should increase expenditure by 3 per cent between the years 1978/79 and 1980/81; during the same period expenditure on the personal social services was planned to fall by 4.7 (pp. 7,11). In such circumstances it is not surprising that, in those areas where domiciliary support for clients with chronic handicaps was seen as a high priority, home nursing services expanded to meet the need and home help services remained static or contracted.

This illustrates clearly how the roles of different services vary across the country, for whilst in some areas home nursing services have been absorbing functions that are traditionally part of the home help service, in others specialist and intensive home help services have been developed with the effect of reducing the range of tasks undertaken by home nurses.

The impact of the home help service on the quality of life and the cost effectiveness of community services depend very largely on the contribution of informal carers. The service must seek a partnership with them as well as with other agencies, both voluntary and statutory, so that an individual package of care is created to meet the needs, not just of the client, but of his family.

Such an approach requires great maturity of judgement on the part of the organiser. When confronted with complex human problems it is tempting to identify and respond to just one part of the matrix without taking into account the thoughts, feelings, and potentialities of all concerned. One of the significant contributions of the Mental Health Act of 1959 was that it brought psychiatrists out of their hospitals and they learned to diagnose whole families instead of viewing the patient in clinical isolation. Similarly, the home help organiser must assess the needs of the family as a whole – not just those of the client – and find solutions that enhance the family's functioning as a caring unit.

Roy Parker (1981 : 23) has pointed out the central dilemma confronting those who provide domiciliary services. On the one hand it is feared that if statutory services assume too many responsibilities, families will opt out 'in an avalanche of abdication', yet if too little help is offered the family 'may collapse under the unrelieved burden'. It is important that, in reaching a decision for an individual client, moral and personal preconceptions about the role of the family are superseded by professional judgements about the actual circumstances that prevail. There is little hard evidence to suggest that families lightly abandon their responsibilities for the sick and infirm; on the contrary, there is much to suggest that families carry impossible burdens. Tizard and Grad (1961) demonstrated that in a significant number of instances family life improved following a patient's admission to hospital.

SOME THEORETICAL CONSIDERATIONS

The first task in developing a professional approach to the assessment of need and the delivery of service is to agree terminology in order to ensure that two home help organisers in the course of discussion mean the same thing when they use the same terms.

Unless common terminology can be agreed to describe key components of the service, discussion remains at a crude and ill-informed level and it is difficult to conceptualise some of the fundamental issues needing debate. When a doctor describes a patient's condition he often gives the diagnosis – he says the patient has tonsillitis, has scarlet fever, or is suffering from appendicitis. A medical diagnosis is a shorthand way of describing a complex situation. Unfortunately, whenever professional groups other than doctors use shorthand words to communicate with one another this is often derided as the use of jargon. Without using shorthand words professional people could hardly communicate intelligently. The jargon words we will use to discuss the policy of the home help service are *extent*, *level*, *cover*, *intensity*, *turnover*, and *complexity*.

There are a variety of ways of expressing the *extent* of the service. It may be calculated in terms of the expenditure devoted to the service in the course of a year; however, figures calculated in this way can be misleading unless it is clear to which year they relate and whether they represent estimates for that year or the actual expenditure. Only if these facts are known can such figures be used reliably to compare the extent of the service in different authorities. Because of the effects of inflation such figures can be confusing if they are used to chart the development of the service over a period of two or more years. A more reliable method is to calculate the number of home helps employed in terms of full-time equivalents. This enables a simple comparison to be made for different years, although when dealing with large numbers over a period of years it must be remembered that improved holiday entitlements and the shorter working week may mean that fewer home help hours are being made available to clients.

Local authorities vary in size, so when comparing the extent to which different authorities rely on the home help service it is best to express the number of home helps as a ratio of the number of people in the total population. However, since the service is predominantly provided for the elderly, a more helpful comparison is to express the number of home helps in terms of 1,000 of the population aged over 65 or 75.

Authorities deploying similar levels of resources may nevertheless follow radically different policies and have different objectives for their services. One authority may spread the service thinly so that large numbers of clients receive a few hours of help each week, whereas another may provide a more intensive service to a small number of clients in very great need. Yet the overall expenditure and the number of hours provided may be the same for each authority.

To understand the relationship between these various elements of the service so that more detailed comparisons can be made of the policies of different authorities, it is helpful to introduce three more terms: first, *level* – the number of hours of home help time which are made available to clients, expressed as the average weekly hours available per 1,000 of the population aged over 65 years; secondly, *cover* – the average weekly cases per 1,000 of the population over 65 years; and thirdly, *intensity* – the average weekly hours provided per client, also expressed in terms of 1,000 of the population over 65 years. It can be seen that:

$$\text{level} = \text{cover} \times \text{intensity}$$

Such a formula gives only a crude indication of differences between the management style of different districts or different authorities but can be used to demonstrate policies in respect of different client groups. For example, an authority may provide a low cover for child care cases but nevertheless offer a high intensity of provision; by contrast, it may offer high cover for the elderly, but low intensity.

The balance between cover and intensity may reflect policy decisions of the authority and arise from firm guidance to organisers; on the other hand, organisers may make their own decisions on these matters and policy may vary from district to district within the same authority, depending on the personality and predilection of each individual organiser. Where this is the case, neither the social services committee nor senior managers may be aware of the actual policy being pursued, since until all the figures are gathered in at the end of the year it is not possible to know what decisions have been made.

It is important that policy makers and managers at all levels are aware of the policy being pursued, so that any changes thought to be desirable can be made, and conscious and positive policies are pursued in conjunction with voluntary organisations and the health service. The way in which increases in budget provision are applied will depend upon the policies to be pursued. For example, a study of the shortfall in existing

Table 5   *Home help services in the south-west 1978–79*

county	level: weekly budget hrs*/1,000 pop.	cover: caseload/ 1,000 elderly	intensity: weekly budget hrs*/case
Avon	266	80	3.3
Gloucestershire	238	66	3.6
Somerset	186	62	3.0
Devon	165	50	3.3
Cornwall	148	46	3.2

*Including travel time and other 'hours' not in home.

services may lead a social services committee to decide that there should be an increase in the intensity of service to clients currently being served. In these circumstances it may be felt possible to keep the number of organisers static and increase the hours of existing home helps; on the other hand, if extended cover is the goal there will be more pressure to match the increase in home helps with more organisers.

Table 5 shows how in 1978/79 the level of service in Gloucestershire was 27 per cent higher than in Somerset but that the cover provided was similar, Gloucestershire deploying its additional resources on intensity. *Table 6* shows that over a three-year period levels of provision changed considerably in the south-west of England. All authorities, including Gloucestershire which decreased its level, increased their cover, but all except Avon reduced the intensity of their provision.

The concepts of level, cover, and intensity enable a picture to be built up of the deployment of home help resources so that comparisons can be made between areas and authorities and over periods of time. However,

Table 6   *Changes in home help services in the south west 1976–79*

county		level	cover	intensity
Avon	1976	250	75	3.3
	1979	266	80	3.3
Gloucestershire	1976	249	62	4.0
	1979	238	66	3.6
Somerset	1976	163	50	3.3
	1979	186	62	3.0
Devon	1976	150	44	3.4
	1979	165	50	3.3
Cornwall	1976	136	39	3.5
	1979	148	46	3.2
percentage change 1976–79				
Avon		+6	+7	0
Gloucestershire		−4	+6	−10
Somerset		+14	+24	−9
Devon		+10	+14	−3
Cornwall		+9	+18	−9

these terms give only a two-dimensional account of the service. Authorities showing identical figures for all three indices may, nevertheless, be offering quite different services if the *turnover* of cases differs markedly. A social services department that concentrates its services on acute needs, such as maternity cases and patients undergoing day surgery, or develops specialist provision enabling early discharge from hospital for certain groups of patients, may have a more rapid turnover of clients than an authority that concentrates its provision on support to clients with long-term physical and mental handicaps. Weekly averages of the number of clients assisted can mask considerable differences in the turnover of clients and in the total number helped during the course of a year.

The sixth jargon word introduced in this chapter is *complexity*. Figures about the service cannot do justice to variations in the quality of provision or differences in the degree of dependency exhibited by clients. Such figures will not reveal that in one area the home help is part of an integrated caring team providing rehabilitation for severely handicapped persons, whereas in another her work is primarily as cook and cleaner. There are not at present any satisfactory measures of complexity. The training of organisers and other staff and the tasks they are expected to perform vary widely, and it will be many years before the growing professionalism of organisers establishes a common approach.

There are differences of view about the relative priority that should be given to different client groups. Depending on the availability of other services and political preferences the proportion of the total service allocated to the elderly, to the mentally ill, to families suspected of child abuse, and other groups, will vary.

The service responds to a variety of personal and social needs. We classify the work into three broad functions, recognising that all three are often undertaken in a single household and that the service centres round the personal relationship between the client and the home help.

(1) *Tending*
   (a) The living environment – assistance to carry out duties necessary to maintain the cleanliness and fabric of the home, including safety and security.
   (b) Food – shopping for food and other household essentials; preparing and cooking meals in the absence of meals-on-wheels or where special dietary or medical requirements make this necessary.
   (c) Warmth – cleaning grates, laying and lighting fires or filling paraffin heaters.
   (d) Personal care – helping clients in and out of bed; to dress and undress. Attending to personal cleanliness, including laundry and emptying commodes.

(2) *Rehabilitation*
   (a) Health – motivating clients to maintain therapy plans set by medical and nursing services, including encouragement in the use of aids to daily living.
   (b) Household management – teaching and advising on nutrition, cooking, budgeting, and the development of household skills.
   (c) Parenting – helping young mothers to provide more effective care for their children.

(3) *Control*
   Assuming direct family responsibilities as, for example, the care of children in the absence of parents or supervising functions in relation to income and expenditure for a mentally handicapped adult living alone.

The task of identifying the differing policies of local authorities from their published statistics is extremely difficult. As we have shown, a given level of provision can be deployed in a great variety of ways, each of which may have its advantages and disadvantages. Furthermore, the allocation of home help hours must be greatly influenced by the type and extent of other services – social work support, community services, day facilities, hospital and residential provision, and standards of housing, all of which vary immensely even within the boundaries of one authority. The nature of family and community support also varies in different localities, and areas with a higher than average number of elderly people in the population, such as the south-west of England and the south coast, must make provision for clients who, in migrating to those areas, have left behind the kinship and community supports that would otherwise sustain them; such factors must affect the way in which domiciliary services are deployed.

No single statement of objectives or policies will suffice for the home help service, either nationally or locally; that is not to say that services should be developed regardless of their impact on social needs and without conscious efforts to set priorities. The resources now deployed and the human needs they are designed to meet are too vast to allow operational decisions to be taken in ignorance of overall objectives, policies, and priorities. Home help managers must engage in a constant dialogue with those employed in related services so that they are familiar with the needs of clients and potential clients and can consider alternative ways of meeting those needs in co-operation with other agencies. Above all, trends in the allocation of the service must be monitored within social services departments so that there can be discussion between managers at all levels about the provision of services and decisions can be taken about the policies to be pursued.

Without such a dialogue using the kind of concepts we have outlined, and without clear statements about the direction in which the service should move, the organiser at local level will feel unsupported; and her day-by-day decisions about the allocation of home help time, instead of following a rational and predetermined pattern, may represent a series of compromises in response to pressures from families, community groups, social workers, general practitioners, hospital consultants, community nurses, and individual politicians. Clear statements of policy and priorities not only assist the organiser at field level to pursue consistent and coherent policies, they enable her to say *No* in the confident knowledge that her decision will be supported by senior managers and, if need be, by the social services committee.

POLICY IN RETROSPECT

Until comparatively recently there has been little study or discussion of the effectiveness of the home help service. Those who work in it have been praised and patronised, and generally the service has been regarded as a valuable adjunct to the care of the elderly and other client groups, but little systematic appraisal has been undertaken on the service to assist in understanding its role in the caring services as a whole; still less have studies examined the potential of the service to provide cost-effective care in a way which is acceptable to recipients.

By recalculating data prepared by Audrey Hunt in her 1976 survey, Bleddyn Davies (1981 : 50) concluded that the intensity of services to clients was too even and did not reflect the varying needs that existed; indeed, he claimed that the proportion of home help clients who were moderately or severely incapacitated fell between 1962 and 1976, and that a significant proportion appeared to be 'neither particularly dependent physically nor socially isolated'. He argued that the service 'seems to run almost independently of local social services management' and that there has been an absence of explicit priorities.

This may represent an over-simplification of a complex problem, for a few paragraphs later the same author draws attention to what he sees as the 'bureaucratisation' of social services departments. In the personal caring services, whether in health or social services, attempts to formulate overall policies and to regulate the use of resources almost invariably lead to accusations of bureaucratic interference and of needless administration. Indeed, even the collection of basic statistical information needed to formulate policies and monitor performance gives rise to such accusations. Since the allocation of resources to individual clients is determined finally by the judgement of practitioners at local level, control from the centre is necessarily tenuous and in many cases can only be achieved over a long period and with the agreement of practitioners. Attempts to restrict the prescription of drugs by medical practitioners have met with this difficulty, as have attempts to ensure that generic social workers devote a greater proportion of their time to clients in minority groups, such as the deaf, the blind, and the mentally ill. Clear and consistent policies can only be developed by an understanding of the overall position and must be transmitted to field staff for consideration and discussion before changes in practice occur.

A study undertaken by the Department of Health and Social Security reviewing national statistical data and research findings concluded that the development of community services had made little impact on the lives of clients with the greatest needs. In considering changes in the balance of care away from long-term hospital and residential accommodation towards care in the community, the study found that 'increases in provision since 1975 have not been geared directly to providing a genuine alternative to those on the margins of institutional care'; and there was 'little if any movement away from long-term hospital or residential care' (1981b : 6,28). This is hardly surprising. Few local authorities have developed positive policies for their domiciliary services. The Department of Health and Social Security has not thought it important enough to include references to concepts such as intensity and cover when promulgating targets for local authorities, but has contented itself with statements about level. Indeed, targets have sometimes been expressed in terms of the number of home helps per head of the population and have disregarded the fact that a more meaningful target would be numbers of home helps per 1,000 of the population over the age of 65.

National figures demonstrate that in the face of increased needs, and even allowing for an improvement in the level of service, cover has been a more highly prized goal than intensity. Figures for England (Appendix 1) show a steady rise in cover and fall in intensity each year since 1972. A case can be made for many more households to receive home help support, but there can be no doubt that priority should be given to those whose needs are greatest and that these clients must be offered an intensity of service which significantly improves their physical and social conditions.

A shift of policy away from extended cover to a more intensive service is not easy to achieve. It requires highly skilled organisers to assess needs, and a home help workforce that is better trained than is general currently. Even before statistical research evidence was widely disseminated, there was an awareness in social services departments of the fact that the intensity of the service was insufficient to prevent admission to hospital or residential care on anything more than a modest scale. For example, Harbert, discussing services in Avon in 1978, said:

> 'There is a wide variation in the number of hours provided but the average hours per week for all clients is 3.2. Clearly, a further extension of the home help service along existing lines will improve the quality of life for more old people and their families, but some concrete proof is needed that the provision of a home help for three or four hours a week will significantly reduce the need for residential care. To achieve such an objective we would need to redeploy the service to ensure that more time is devoted to a smaller number of households where the need is greatest, and to provide services in the evenings and at weekends (which are difficult and expensive to staff). This would be an important change of policy.'
> (1978 : 27)

As shown in Chapter 3, since the middle 1970s there has been a marked increase in special schemes under which intensive and specialist services are provided for clients with the greatest needs. These schemes often arrange up to twenty-four hours of cover, including weekend work, enabling early discharge from hospital and avoiding the need for admission. Usually special training is provided for the workforce. Statistics about such services are not always included in returns about the home help service so intensity of provision across the country may be higher than the official home help returns have indicated.

A study of clients admitted to elderly persons' homes and homes for the elderly mentally infirm in Avon (Avon Social Services Department 1980) showed that, when asked whether the provision of domiciliary services would avoid the need for admission, social workers put forward alternatives for 50 per cent of the clients. Where alternatives were mentioned the services suggested most frequently were those most prevalent: home helps, mobile meals, and sheltered housing. The home help service was listed more frequently than any other service. Avon provides a more intensive home help service than many authorities and also has a home aide service, providing specialist and intensive help for those in greatest need; it is, therefore, likely that studies elsewhere would produce similar results or show an even greater shortfall of home help provision. This may demonstrate the need for an extension of these services but it could also signify that existing provision is not allocated to the best advantage. Other research has shown that applicants for residential care have received little or no support from domiciliary services and that their capacity to carry out domestic tasks may be unknown at the time of admission.

Although intensive home help provision can reduce the need for hospital or residential care, the shortage of available resources makes it necessary for organisers continually to review the allocation of the service. Intensive help which serves only to delay admission to hospital or a home for several weeks may not be the most constructive use of home help time. On the other hand, if domiciliary services can enable a patient to leave hospital at an earlier date than would otherwise be possible, this may help to avoid some of the ill-effects of hospital care and speed the patient's full recovery and rehabilitation. Similarly, intensive care at home may make it unnecessary for a client to enter hospital, so minimising the extent of his personal trauma and ensuring that he is kept in familiar surroundings in which rehabilitation has the best chance of success. The availability of emergency services outside normal office hours and an organisational system that permits the deployment of intensive services for short periods can, if properly managed, offer immense benefits.

Nevertheless, home help provision is but one of a number of services for which social services committees are responsible. Even when there is an immense pressure on the home help service the committee will need to decide whether any increased funds which can be made available should be allocated to the service, or whether better value will be obtained by appointing more social workers, extending meals-on-wheels, providing day care services, or building more residential homes.

It should not be assumed that the home help service, if provided in sufficient quantity, can enable every client with a chronic medical or mental condition to remain at home. With good co-operation between the home help service and informal carers, as well as other service providers, much more can be done to support people in their own homes, but not only is intensive home care very expensive -- sometimes more expensive than residential care when all the costs are taken into account -- it may still prove inadequate to meet the needs of some clients.

To be helpful, statements of policy about the home help service must be readily understandable to managers at all levels in the social services department, to clients and to staff in the health and personal social services who request assistance. If the criteria for the allocation of home help time are widely known and understood the task of organisers will be considerably eased, since requests for assistance will be more appropriate and false expectations are less likely to be aroused.

SUGGESTED OPERATIONAL CRITERIA

High-sounding phrases used to discuss the service, its policies, and its practices must be translated by field organisers into criteria for action. Statements of aims and purposes must mean the same thing to committee members and managers at all levels, or policy is merely an illusion. Written statements are of themselves insufficient to ensure a coherent and unified policy within the service; they are the basis for understanding the issues involved and for promoting discussion.

Within broad policies established for the service in each authority there must be room for flexibility and for organisers to make judgements about how the needs of individual clients can best be met. There must be sufficient delegation to enable an appropriate service to be offered in different geographical areas with contrasting needs. Policy statements are like cairns of stones in the Highlands -- they indicate the direction the traveller must take but do not specify the track; provided he uses them as his guide the wayfarer will not lose his way or fall into a crevasse.

Traditionally, the service has concentrated on the tending role -- the provision of a clean home, food, warmth, and personal care -- which requires a few hours each week of home help time. Other functions -- rehabilitation and control -- require more skill and must generally be provided on a more intensive basis. The allocation of a service to care for a family of children may make it necessary to withdraw services from ten households requiring help with tending tasks. For this reason, a policy must be promulgated at a senior level in each authority about the relative priority that is to be offered to rehabilitation and control activity, as opposed to those households where tending is the main service to be provided. This may be a matter which elected members will wish to decide.

Sometimes policies can best be achieved by creating teams of staff to specialise in particular areas of work. This enables appropriate skills to be developed; eases relationships with specialist social work, medical, and nursing staff; and ensures that an agreed level of provision is made available for a particular range of duties, such as child abuse work or the rehabilitation of psychiatrically ill mothers.

Whether the organisation of the service is based on specialist or generic teams of home helps, guidance must be given on the cover and intensity that should be provided in respect of tending, rehabilitative, and control tasks. It will, for example, be reasonable to specify the total number of hours per year that local organisers will be permitted to allocate to the long-term care of children. Should an organiser wish to extend these hours she will be required to discuss the position with senior colleagues who, if they agree with her judgement, will seek to increase the number of hours available to her, or will ensure that discussions take place with other professional staff in the locality about the reduction of service that will occur in other areas of activity. Each year the relative priority given to different categories of need should be redefined in consultation with all the interested parties.

Within those households where the prime function of the service relates to tending, it is necessary for organisers to determine priorities. The following schedule has been found helpful in the County of Avon.

Priority 1 – where daily help is required in connection with personal care, warmth, *and* food.

Priority 2 – where daily help is required under *one* of the categories listed in priority 1.

Priority 3 – where help is required on several days of the week in connection with personal care, warmth, *and* food.

Priority 4 – where help is required on several days of the week in connection with *one* of the categories mentioned in priority 3.

Priority 5 – where extreme hardship is likely to result if the service is refused or withdrawn; this group includes families where child abuse is known or suspected.

These priorities assume that, except in special circumstances – for example, to provide relief for relatives – services will not be provided where an able-bodied relative is available and willing to assist the client. It will be noted that such a classification of priorities implies that intensity will take precedence over cover.

7 · The employment framework

Since the middle of the 1960s major legislative changes have been made affecting the rights of employees and the obligations of employers in the United Kingdom. These changes have had a significant impact on the home help service and the way in which it is managed. Whereas previously a home help organiser required little knowledge of employment law she must now have a detailed understanding of complex legislation. It is likely that in many authorities the law is imperfectly understood by managers and workforce alike, and that because the home help service is not highly unionised this goes unnoticed and unremarked.

Responsibility for operating the service within the law rests with the local authority and, except in relation to a limited range of duties, not on individual organising staff. Many matters will be the subject of authority-wide procedures laid down by a personnel or finance department, whilst other procedures will be covered by guidance from within the social services department. Nevertheless, because the home help service is a substantial employer, much responsibility rests with individual organisers to ensure that legal responsibilities are met and that employees receive all the protection to which they are entitled. A failure in this respect can bring severe penalties to the local authority.

A number of major pieces of legislation govern relationships between employer and employee. The main enactments are listed below and are described in the text that follows. The law in relation to employment changes so regularly that no account can be considered to be exhaustive, and readers are advised to assume that what follows will not remain up-to-date in every detail for more than a few months. It should be noted that some of the legislation has been repealed, modified, or consolidated by later Acts of Parliament.

Contracts of Employment Acts 1963–72
Redundancy Payments Act 1965–69
Equal Pay Act 1970
Industrial Relations Act 1971
Health and Safety at Work Act 1974
Rehabilitation of Offenders Act 1974
Trade Union and Labour Relations Act 1974
Sex Discrimination Act 1975
Employment Protection Act 1975
Trade Union and Labour Relations (Amendment) Act 1976
Race Relations Act 1976
Employment Protection (Consolidation) Act 1978
Employment Act 1980
Employment Act 1982

COLLECTIVE BARGAINING

Employees are entitled to join an independent trade union. They are also entitled to have time off for trade union activities approved by their employer and reasonable time off to carry out trade union duties. New employees should have their attention drawn to these entitlements, although the scattered labour force which makes up the home help service together with the fact that the overwhelming majority of home helps are part-time employees make it difficult for trade unions to recruit and organise these staff. Space on a notice board facilitates communications between trade unions and their members but it is difficult to ensure that home helps have regular access to the material displayed.

Trade union representatives are entitled to reasonable office facilities to carry out their duties; this primarily means the use of a telephone and photocopying equipment. Problems of divided loyalties may prevent a home help from asking for time off to carry out trade union duties; she may know that there is no spare capacity available and that a morning spent on trade union work will mean that a client goes without a service. Such problems can be overcome or minimised by careful planning and by the home help making her request for time off well in advance of the event.

The Registrar of Friendly Societies maintains a list of trade unions and employers' associations. An organisation can be removed from the list if its rules do not comply with those laid down by the Trade Union and Labour Relations Act of 1974. The rules mainly concern the keeping of proper records and accounts. An employing authority has a duty to disclose to representatives of trade unions information necessary for collective bargaining.

A few authorities have closed shop agreements by which the employer requires each employee within an identifiable class to become a member of the union or one of the unions which is, or are, parties to the agreement. The importance of such an agreement is that an employee who is subject to it will lose his job if for any reason he leaves the union or is expelled from it. The conditions of union membership agreements have been modified by the Employment Act of 1980 by protecting employees who are not union members at the time of the agreement and those who object to union membership on grounds of conscience or political conviction. A person who is, or is seeking to be, in employment where there is a union membership agreement can complain to an industrial tribunal that he has been unreasonably excluded or expelled from the union. The tribunal can order the union to take a person into, or back into, membership and award compensation. All union membership agreements must now be approved by a ballot of relevant employees.

Agreements between trade unions and employers may be made locally or nationally, that is, between an employer and local union representatives or between a group representing employers nationally and trade unions. An agreement is not legally enforceable unless it is in writing and contains provisions stating that the parties intend that it shall be a legally enforceable contract. A collective agreement between a trade union and employer can include a clause specifying that the employee will not strike. This can only be effective if appropriate wording is included in the contract of employment of each individual employee.

Pay and conditions of service for home helps are determined in the United Kingdom by the National Joint Council for Local Authorities' Services (Manual Workers) which covers over 1 million personnel. The joint council comprises representatives from relevant trade unions and local authority associations. The National Joint Council for Administrative, Professional, Technical and Clerical Services deals with the pay and conditions of service for most local authority 'white collar' staff outside schools and colleges; local authorities select salary levels for home help organisers from the variety of grades agreed by this joint council.

The Advisory, Conciliation and Arbitration Service is an important statutory body set up by the Employment Protection Act of 1975 and it can be consulted by either party to a dispute as a means of assisting in its resolution. In the event of a serious dispute arising involving the home help service, organisers would find it helpful to familiarise themselves with the law relating to picketing and secret ballots.

CONTRACTS

Every employee is entitled to receive a written statement of particulars about his employment not less than thirteen weeks after taking up the post. The statement must include (1) the scale or rate of remuneration; (2) the intervals at which remuneration is paid; (3) the terms and conditions relating to hours of work; (4) terms and conditions relating to (a) entitlement to holidays including public holidays and holiday pay, (b) entitlement to payment during periods of sickness and accident, (c) entitlement to pensions and pension contributions; (5) steps to be followed in any grievance which an employee might have; (6) the date on which a fixed term contract is to end; (7) information about the calculation of accrued holiday pay due on termination of employment; (8) the job title of the employee's occupation; (9) any disciplinary rules; and (10) the name of the person the employee can petition if he is not satisfied with any disciplinary decision relating to him.

The fact that the hours of work must be stated in the contract of employment has caused problems for the home help service, especially in rural areas. Within the overall budget provision, organisers attempt to vary the hours of home helps. As demand for the service changes, a particular home help may agree to increase her hours to cover the temporary sickness of a colleague, to take on additional work, or to increase the number of hours she currently provides to her own clients; the organiser must issue an amended statement of particulars in such instances. If, at a later date, the additional hours are no longer required the contract must be re-negotiated; but the home help may not wish to revert to her former hours and the organiser may be required to find additional work for her. This can pose serious difficulties in sparsely populated areas where it may be necessary for a home help to travel many miles in order to continue working her contracted hours. Employment may be offered for a temporary period provided this is made clear at the outset.

Problems also arise where the organiser seeks to reduce the service in the summer in order to have extra budgetary provision in the winter months. If she engages additional hours to carry out firelighting in the winter she may face claims for unfair dismissal when she is unable to find work for her home helps in the summer.

Casual employment suited the domestic circumstances of a great many women whose talents are now largely lost to the service. It was often the practice for home helps to decide that when a client went into hospital or died they would take a few weeks' break, returning to work at a later date, possibly working different hours. Now every change must be properly documented, with gaps in service being recorded as periods of unpaid leave, applications for which must be made in some authorities to an officer of the personnel department for approval.

In reducing opportunities for casual employment, legislation has made the home help service less flexible and less responsive to local needs, and made it more difficult for housewives to undertake a few weeks of casual work while their children are at school. It is possible to overcome the inflexibility of the law to some extent in respect of employees who are prepared to work for less than sixteen hours a week, but it can be uneconomic to employ part-time staff unless they work for well over fourteen hours a week because of the national insurance contributions payable on their behalf. There are also formidable administrative problems for the organiser if her workforce is made up of large numbers of staff working only a few hours a week each. It can be argued that the effective development of the service demands a stable and reliable workforce composed of trained staff, and employment legislation has done much to bring this about.

Contracts of employment serve as a protection to employer and employee alike. An employee may refuse to undertake duties that are not specified in the written particulars supplied. If she carries out work not in her job description she may have a case, under national agreements between local authorities and trade unions, to apply for increased remuneration. Organisers must be wary about asking staff to volunteer for, or accept, additional duties, since this can cause wage drift; managers in some authorities have been threatened with disciplinary action if they allow this to occur. However, changes in the service, including local experimentation, cannot proceed naturally and smoothly within the straightjacket of rigid job descriptions; some flexibility in working arrangement is necessary to meet changing circumstances.

Pension arrangements create additional problems for the organiser who wishes to use her workforce flexibly. Contributory pensions apply to employees who work for thirty hours per week or more. Thus some home helps wish to work more than thirty hours in order to secure a pension, whilst others endeavour to work less than thirty hours to avoid making contributions. Yet others move from one status to the other, creating considerable work for the authority in adjusting their statement of particulars and their contribution record. Problems have arisen when organisers and home helps studying for the Diploma in Home Help Organisation seek to reduce their working hours but do not wish to lose the benefits of superannuated service.

Employees are entitled to an itemised pay statement. This has proved extremely helpful in the home help service as pay arrangements can be complex, with premium payments, additional hours, sickness deductions, and other adjustments often made several weeks after the event to which they relate. Employees are also entitled to a guaranteed payment of wages if their contract is for more than three months and they work for more than sixteen hours per week (eight hours if over five years' service). This has proved very inconvenient for the management of services. When a client dies, goes into hospital, or for some other reason ceases to require a service, the home help is usually allocated to another client, but there may be some delay in making or notifying these arrangements which means that the home help will be paid for doing nothing – something that could provoke public criticism for the authority.

DISMISSALS AND REDUNDANCY

An employee who works for more than sixteen hours per week is entitled to receive from one week's notice of dismissal after one month of continuous service, rising to three months' notice after twelve years' service. She is also entitled to a written statement giving the reasons for her dismissal. An employee who works between eight and sixteen hours per week is entitled to similar protection after five years' service. The employer can insist upon one week's notice from his employee unless the contract of employment specifies otherwise.

Provisions relating to unfair dismissal have been refined in several pieces of legislation. An employee who feels that he has been unfairly dismissed has the right to state his case before an industrial tribunal, provided he has over one year's service and works a minimum of sixteen hours per week (eight hours if over five years' service). This protection does not extend to men over 65 or women over 60 years.

Misconduct by an employee outside his employment can lead to dismissal if it seriously affects the performance of his job. Views and practices differ widely, and it is wise for organisers to acquaint themselves of the likely attitude of elected representatives before embarking on the dismissal of an employee for offences or other actions committed whilst off duty. If she feels strongly, an organiser may be willing to dismiss an employee even though she knows that, on appeal to elected representatives, the employee is likely to be reinstated. However, her reputation and that of the service cannot afford to have too many disagreements of this kind.

Dismissal following disciplinary procedures mostly relates to the falsification of time sheets, and this is sometimes encouraged by clients who are prepared to sign for a service they have not received because they wish to show their appreciation. Opportunities for dishonesty are great; managers must be aware of this and carefully monitor the performance of their staff. Auditor staff should be asked to investigate irregularities as soon as they are discovered.

The formalities that now surround engagement and dismissal are in sharp contrast to the position in previous years, when a home help might be offered a few hours of work on a casual basis with no contract. A home help whose work was poor, or whose time-keeping was unsatisfactory, would be warned and, if no improvement ensued, would simply be given no more work. Similarly, a home help who was sick might be given notice so that the organiser could engage a replacement. The sick home help might return to her employment in due course, but the employer had no obligation towards her.

An employee can appeal to an industrial tribunal against unfair dismissal as soon as notice of dismissal is received and up to three months after dismissal has become effective. It is unfair to dismiss an employee for exercising his right to become a member of, or be active in, a trade union. In certain circumstances an employee may be able successfully to claim constructive dismissal if he can convince an industrial tribunal that his employer's conduct was such that he was entitled to terminate his own employment.

An employee is entitled to be told the reasons for his or her dismissal and may be accompanied by a trade union official or solicitor at a disciplinary hearing. A home help may appeal against a decision to dismiss her, in which case a sub-committee of elected members will review the matter and require evidence to satisfy themselves that the organiser has just grounds for her actions. If the appeal is upheld, or if it eventually reaches an industrial tribunal and is upheld, the organiser may be required to absorb the home help into her workforce again.

Special provisions apply where an employer contracts his workforce on the grounds that the need for employees to undertake work of a particular kind has diminished or ceased. It would be extremely difficult for a local authority to demonstrate that social needs had diminished to the extent that it could make home helps redundant. Nevertheless, where financial restrictions force local authorities to reduce expenditure quickly it can be necessary to dismiss staff, and a number of social services departments have been faced with the need to make staff redundant. In these circumstances employees are entitled by law to redundancy payments calculated on the basis of continuous service, provided that they have worked for more than two years, are under pensionable age, and work for more than sixteen hours a week (or eight if for more than five years).

Certain formalities are required before redundancy payments are payable. The employer must consult with recognised trade unions prior to dismissal taking effect. If over a hundred people are to be made redundant, consultation must take place at least ninety days in advance, but where between ten and ninety-nine people are affected the minimum consultation period is thirty days. Employees facing redundancy are entitled to have time off work to look for alternative employment or training.

Whilst it is rare for local authorities to invoke redundancy payments legislation, there are occasions when it may be advantageous for an employee to claim that his dismissal from the service is caused by redundancy; he may then apply to an industrial tribunal to the effect that, since the authority has not followed the correct procedure, he has been unfairly dismissed. This possibility arises in the home help service when arrangements are made for a member of staff to carry out specified work. For example, a home help may care for a family of children for a period in excess of two years; when the children grow up, or a parent returns to the household, the home help may be entitled to redundancy pay unless her contract of employment permits her to be transferred to other forms of work.

Other examples of situations that have presented difficulties in relation to the Redundancy Payments Act include the allocation of a home help to support day-care staff at meal times with a multi-handicapped client and long-term assistance to a thalidomide young man attending college. In such cases the contract of employment must be specific about the nature of the duties, but there can be no certainty that these precise duties will continue to be required indefinitely.

During a time when a local authority is reducing manpower it is important that opportunities are provided for displaced employees to be offered vacant posts that arise in other sections and other departments of the authority. It may become necessary to suspend normal arrangements for recruiting home helps, clerks, and organisers to ensure that vacancies are first offered to staff at risk. Whilst this can cause delays, particularly if there are many staff concerned who require time to consider their positions, it is unavoidable and the service may suffer in the short term as a result. Changes and reductions in the school meals service during recent years have led to a number of redeployment exercises of this kind, although the size and flexibility of the home help budget usually means that new staff can be absorbed in great numbers on the understanding that natural wastage over a period will reduce any temporary over-staffing. Few authorities employ relief or peripatetic staff to cover vacancies of organisers and clerks. A scattered workforce demands consistent management, and staff morale suffers when long periods elapse during which management posts are not filled.

Employees must be permitted reasonable time off to perform duties connected with certain public offices. Such duties include membership of a health, local, or water authority; jury service; service of justice of the peace; membership of the managing or governing body of a maintained educational establishment; and membership of a statutory tribunal.

DISCRIMINATION

The law no longer allows employers a free hand in the way in which they select their employees, and restrictions are imposed to ensure that certain types of employee who may otherwise be disadvantaged do not suffer discrimination. The main groups protected are women, including pregnant women, handicapped or sick persons, ex-offenders, and racial minorities.

The Sex Discrimination Act of 1975 made sex discrimination unlawful in employment; training; education; the provision of goods, facilities, and services; and in the disposal and management of premises. It affords protection against discrimination to both men and women (and against married persons) and extends to indirect discrimination, by which the terms and conditions that are laid down ensure that only persons of a particular sex can comply with them. All employers with more than five employees are covered by the legislation.

Certain exceptions are made to the general application of the legislation where it can be shown that a person's sex is a genuine occupational qualification. There are a number of these exceptions, such as where physiology is important, in the modelling of clothes or in dramatic performances. Some of the exceptions are relevant to the home help service and it is important that managers in the service are aware of them.

A genuine occupational qualification exists where it can be shown that considerations of decency or privacy require the post to be held specifically by a man or woman because of the likelihood of physical contact, or where people may be present in a state of undress. An organiser may therefore legitimately transfer a male home help from a household where a confused female needs personal attention or is liable to wander without clothes. It is also possible to argue that a particular task involves the provision of personal services promoting welfare and education, and that a person of a particular sex is more likely to achieve the desired response; for example, it would be inappropriate to provide a male home help to a woman who is frightened of men, and vice versa.

The employer may decide that it is necessary for the job holder to live on the premises but, because there is no separate sleeping or sanitary accommodation, it is unreasonable for the work to be undertaken by an employee of a particular sex; this may arise in a single-sex establishment or in a single-sex part of an establishment. Restrictions are sometimes placed upon residential home help provision because of the absence of suitable sleeping arrangements.

A person who feels discriminated against may make a complaint even though he or she did not apply for the job. It is unlawful to offer different terms or conditions of service in relation to the sex of the applicant. Once in employment, it is illegal to discriminate between the sexes in affording access to training, promotion, or other benefits, facilities, or services. There are some exceptions relating to retirement and pregnancy.

The Sex Discrimination Act of 1975 established the Equal Opportunities Commission which can enquire into complaints. Complaints can also be taken to an industrial tribunal. Since home helps are employed to promote the welfare of clients it is lawful for an organiser to deploy a mixed workforce of men and women in a discriminatory way. She will be contravening the law, however, if she refuses to appoint men on the basis that male home helps are unsuitable. Clients sometimes discriminate, specifying that they do not wish a man to be allocated to them. Since it is important to ensure a compatibility between the client and the home help, the wishes of clients in this matter are very important and should be observed wherever possible. Advertisements for organisers' posts are increasingly attracting male applicants, and this poses some difficulties for a service that is predominantly female-orientated. It may be felt that an organiser who must visit clients, many of them women, and ask intimate personal questions, needs to be particularly understanding and sensitive; perhaps the criterion in this regard for selecting male organisers is more rigorously applied than it is for females. Then, too, the male organiser must work with a largely female workforce, with a team of colleague organisers who are also mostly female; he may also be accountable to a woman – something that some men find difficult. When interviewing male applicants, experience, personality, training, and aptitude must be taken into account, and a judgement made about their suitability for undertaking the job; provided it can be shown that a male applicant is rejected on grounds of his unsuitability and not on grounds of his sex, the selection process is likely to be within the law.

It may be considered that many authorities discriminate against women in the home help service by the limited opportunities given to such staff for promotion and training. The law has not been particularly successful in opening up employment prospects for women, who are still to be found in large numbers in low-paid occupations and at relatively low levels on the promotional ladder. Compared with jobs carrying similar responsibilities even within social services departments, the home help organiser is generally poorly paid; this arises because it has been predominantly a female occupation and because promotion and training opportunities for this group of staff have been severely limited. A cynic might argue that the home help service is living proof that the Sex Discrimination Act has failed.

Under the Equal Pay Act of 1970 it is illegal to discriminate on grounds of sex with regard to pay and terms and conditions of employment. Section 1 of the Act provides for equal treatment for men and women where they are engaged in the same or broadly similar work, or where a woman's job has been rated as equivalent to a man's job through job evaluation or some other exercise, even though the nature of the job is different. Section 2 places the onus of proof on the employer to show, in cases of dispute, that the differences in the terms and conditions of employment of the woman who is claiming equal treatment with the man are genuinely due to material differences between her case and his. Section 3 of the Equal Pay Act refers to collective agreements; if these contain discriminatory clauses they may be reported to the Advisory, Conciliation and Arbitration Service. Provision was made in the early 1970s for the then different rates of pay for male and female home helps to be assimilated to one grade. In authorities where organisers are particularly badly paid Section 3 of the Equal Pay Act is being cited as a reason why they should be regraded.

Women cannot be dismissed on grounds of pregnancy; they must be given paid time off for antenatal care and have certain rights in respect of returning to work after the birth of a baby. To exercise these rights, women wishing to return after confinement must give written notice of their intention prior to leaving, and provide their employers with three weeks' notice of the actual date of their return. In some circumstances an employer may offer a returning woman not her original job but another suitable alternative post. The uncertainties about whether and when a pregnant home help will return to her job make it difficult to plan services, and there can be friction when a returning home help finds that her clients have got used to a new home help and she is placed elsewhere.

The Rehabilitation of Offenders Act of 1974 provides that in certain circumstances ex-offenders no longer have to reveal a criminal record to prospective employers. An employer who refuses to engage or dismisses a rehabilitated person on the grounds of his criminal record can be required to answer to an industrial tribunal. Certain posts in social services departments are exempt from the effects of the Act – including home helps. Requests for references in connection with applications for posts should contain a clause to this effect. When giving a reference for an employee who has committed an offence, managers should satisfy themselves whether or not the Rehabilitation of Offenders Act applies.

The Race Relations Act of 1976 was drawn up on the same basis as the Sex Discrimination Act and makes racial discrimination unlawful in employment, training, education, and in the provision of goods. The Act strengthens the definition of racial discrimination to include indirect discrimination and extends its definition to include victimisation. It specifies where membership of a particular racial group can be said to be a genuine occupational qualification for a post.

Individual managers are personally liable – along with their employers – for acts of racial discrimination that they knowingly commit. However, the Act provides for limited positive discrimination in favour of particular racial groups. The Council for Racial Equality is a statutory body whose duties include the investigation of complaints of racial discrimination. Individual complaints from employees can also be made to an industrial tribunal.

In inner city areas with high levels of unemployment, the powers contained in the Act to discriminate positively in favour of particular racial groups can be used to create worthwhile employment for the disadvantaged. Whilst a home help organiser will wish to comply with the law, she will be faced with clients who are unwilling to receive assistance from home helps drawn from another racial group. This is particularly so of the elderly, who find it difficult to accept the customs and habits of home helps from different cultural backgrounds.

HEALTH AND SAFETY AT WORK

The home help service was not covered by a statutory code of practice for health and safety until the implementation of the Health and Safety at Work Act of 1974. Throughout the nineteenth and twentieth centuries a series of Acts of Parliament regulated working conditions in those workplaces where ill-health and accident were a serious hazard – particularly factories, mines, and quarries. More recently agriculture was included, and in 1963 the Offices, Shops and Railway Premises Act brought large numbers of white-collar workers into the ambit of health and welfare legislation. However, despite about thirty statutes there were still an estimated 5–6 million workers outside statutory provision of any kind when the Robens Committee reported on health and safety at work in 1972. Whilst home help organisers and their clerks had protection under the Offices, Shops and Railway Premises Act, there was no requirement on employers to ensure that home helps were advised about health hazards or officially instructed about safety problems.

The Robens Committee undertook a comprehensive examination of health and safety provision. Apart from recommending a new statutory framework that would include all workplaces and workpeople within health and safety regulations, the committee argued that improvements in work practices could not depend on negative regulation by external agencies. It stressed the need for a new style of safety organisation that would include workpeople themselves as well as management and so produce a self-regulating system, less dependent on threat and exhortation from outside.

The principles outlined by the Robens Committee were the basis of the Health and Safety at Work Act of 1974. The obscure wording of the Act at first led many people to believe that the home help service was excluded from its provisions; this arose because, although Section 1 states that the Act applies to all people *at work*, Section 51 makes an exception for domestic servants in private households. However, in 1978 the Health and Safety Executive ruled that, along with a number of other categories of people who work in premises not under the control of their employer, home helps were indeed included in the main provisions of the Act.

The Act is expressed in general terms covering all forms of employment, including many previously outside statutory control, such as the home help service, schools, libraries, residential establishments, and rent collection. The employer has a duty to provide a safe working environment so far as it is reasonably practicable to do so. Employers must also supply information to employees on matters affecting their health and safety, and arrange instruction, training, and supervision for employees. The training and instruction must relate not merely to the health and safety of the employee but also to that of other persons who may be affected in the workplace. It is not enough for home helps to be made aware of the hazards they may encounter and of how to handle them; they must be aware of the need to protect others. For example, they must take care to ensure that a hot iron or boiling saucepan is out of reach of a child, and they must ensure that the trailing lead of a vacuum cleaner is not a hazard to a handicapped or frail old person; if they are aware of an appliance in a faulty condition they must not use it and they must draw the fault to the attention of the householder.

A responsibility rests on every employer to issue a statement setting out a safety policy and to describe the organisational arrangements for carrying it out. In a large organisation like a local authority with a very wide range of functions it is not practicable for one policy statement to cover each function in sufficient detail. It is therefore usual for local authorities to issue a safety policy for the organisation as a whole, together with a separate statement in relation to the social services department and a further specific statement for the home help service. The purpose of such statements, which should be prominently displayed, is to ensure that staff at all levels clearly understand their responsibilities. The Health and Safety Executive has suggested that the main hazards that might be encountered should be listed in the policy statement.

The Robens Committee underlined the need to involve the workforce if there were to be a greater awareness of safety issues. The Act therefore makes provision for trade unions to appoint safety representatives to represent employees in consultations with the employer on matters of safety. The safety representative is empowered to undertake inspections, including accident investigations, to have access to relevant documents, and to make representations to the employer. The employer is required to provide time off with pay for these duties. Safety representatives have no right of entry to the workplaces of home helps; consequently their role is very limited. Where safety representatives make a request, the employer is obliged to create a safety committee with representatives of employees and management to discuss issues of mutual concern, to consider policy, identify hazards, and study analyses of accidents.

It is important that the safety policy of the service specifies the responsibilities of home help organisers for instructing and informing home helps. The Act places an obligation on employers to provide 'such information, instruction, training and supervision as is necessary to ensure as far as is reasonably practical the health and safety at work of his employees'. It is therefore necessary for new home helps to be given some basic information very soon after the start of their employment – preferably on the first day. In particular, home helps must be aware of (a) the major risks associated with the job and how to minimise them, (b) the accident reporting procedure, (c) procedures to be followed in the event of emergencies, and (d) the hazard reporting procedure (where the home help identifies a risk that he or she is unable to eradicate).

The home help service has experienced great difficulty in operating the provisions of health and safety legislation. The homes of the elderly and handicapped and those of families in poor circumstances often contain worn fabric, furniture, and equipment. Organisers cannot demand that all defective items are replaced; they can, however, with persuasion, be sure that unsafe floorcoverings are removed or more firmly fixed, and in some circumstances may feel it reasonable to ensure that assistance is provided from statutory or voluntary funds to install safe cooking and heating appliances. Elderly people become attached to items of furniture and equipment that have been in their possession for many years and are likely to resent any suggestion that the organiser is carrying out an inspection.

Dangerous bannister rails, unsafe windows, broken floorboards, and defective electrical wiring may be the responsibility of the landlord. He may be unwilling to undertake the repairs felt to be essential by the organiser, or, if he can be persuaded to act, he may increase the rent, causing distress to the client. Legislation has focused attention on the health and safety hazards for home helps and has made managers and the home helps themselves more aware of the need to provide a safe working environment. Some compromises are inevitable, however; when gentle persuasion does not succeed it will be prudent to continue the service despite the hazards. Where the law permits a dwelling to be occupied by a client it would be difficult to argue that it is too unsafe for a home help.

The work of a home help is not without its own dangers; the increasing proportion of personal caring functions now carried out makes home helps particularly vulnerable to muscle strain and back injury. In Avon in 1980 home helps suffered more back injury at work than any other occupational group employed by the county council. Nearly 3 per cent reported back injuries during the course of the year. A study carried out in Stockholm during 1977 showed that one in eight pensioners with a home help received considerable lifting assistance (International Council of Home Help Services 1980 : 21). Special lifting equipment was rarely available, and over half the home helps reported some disorders of the musculo-skeletal system. It was thought that the recruitment of more men would be desirable and that more staff should work in pairs. Doubtless similar results would be found from studies in the United Kingdom. This indicates the need for special instruction to home helps and the provision of adequate equipment.

The Local Government Training Board has issued material composed of notes and slides that cover the basic training requirements for home helps in relation to health and safety matters; these are extensively used by social services departments. In 1980 the National Council of Home Help Services undertook a survey to discover the extent to which authorities provided home helps with written information about their responsibilities in relation to health and safety (National Council of Home Help Services 1981). Of forty-eight authorities replying to a questionnaire, thirty-four indicated that written information *was* supplied to home helps; a further seven authorities indicated that written information was in the course of preparation. On the whole the material was assembled separately in booklet or leaflet form, but in some instances it was combined with information about terms and conditions of service and operational information made available to employees at the start of their employment. A working party of the National Council recommended that guideline notes on health and safety matters should be issued to home helps, that this information should be separate from other general employment information, and that it should be specifically designed and produced for home helps.

CONCLUSIONS

Nationally, the ratio of organisers to home helps has changed little in a ten-year period, but it is clear that employment legislation has added significant burdens to organisers and their clerks. Inevitably the management of the bureaucratic system takes priority over care. As staff become more aware of their rights, administrative pressure on organisers will become even greater. In many authorities organisers are the lowest graded staff who interview and appoint staff; frequently they carry out their duties with the minimum supervision, and it is therefore essential that they have adequate training and a full grasp of employment law and its implications.

There can be no doubt that the impact of legislative change has been very great on the workload of organisers and on the style of management under which the service operates. Organisers have been required to be more careful in selecting staff. They cannot afford to take chances with a doubtful employee because not only may it prove difficult to effect a dismissal but such a course is likely to be unpleasant and prove very time-consuming. The organiser who decides to embark on dismissal for a member of her staff will be required to keep full records showing how the employee has performed and indicating precisely what work has not been done or has been done badly, and the dates and times when warnings have been given. She may be required to show that, having noted the deficiencies in the home help, she has attempted to provide training or other instruction to overcome them. Local authorities, like other employers, are reluctant to risk defending themselves before an industrial tribunal; consequently, home help organisers and other managers in social services departments are sometimes expected to tolerate incompetence and misconduct much longer than they would like.

Failure by an organiser to comply with employment legislation may bring a sharp reaction from trade unions and invoke enquiries by senior staff from two or three departments, possibly leading to a report to elected members. Large organisations like local authorities build a strong protective wall between themselves and outside investigating bodies such as the district auditor, industrial tribunals, and the Ombudsman. It is in their nature for local authorities to be sensitive to public criticism, especially when it emanates from an impartial and statutory body.

Errors of judgement or incompetence by an organiser in assessing the needs of clients and allocating resources are difficult to detect, and no powerful organisation exists to make an effective challenge to local authorities on matters other than expenditure, employment procedures, and administration. It is therefore incumbent on social services to ensure that there is good professional direction and a built-in capacity to monitor the quality of the service provided. Administrative procedures and data collection processes designed to enable central departments to be satisfied that the service is operating within the law, and within laid-down manpower and financial controls, must be organised in a way that does not unduly restrict the ability of staff to respond quickly and flexibly to need.

In approving the complex series of Acts of Parliament covering employment issues Parliament was certainly unaware of their cumulative cost. Each Act is unexceptionable in its aims and aspirations, but each Act has its price in terms of limiting the flexibility of services, adding to administrative burdens, increasing direct costs, and permitting staff to absent themselves from their primary tasks on full pay. The sum total of additional costs for the home help service are not known, but direct comparisons of numbers of staff in the service between 1972 and now represent a considerable overstatement of the actual growth achieved by the service in this time.

8 · Assessment and
review of
individual needs

The home help service is a costly resource and except in rare circumstances the client does not meet the full cost by direct payment. The rates and taxes that largely pay for the service are drawn from the community generally, and every member of the public has a right to receive a service based on his needs within the resources available; this applies whether the service is provided by a statutory body or an independent organisation with government subsidies. There are only two legitimate ways of allocating public resources. The first is for elected representatives to make decisions on behalf of the community; the second is by the exercise of a professional judgement based on knowledge and skill. That is not to say that a professional judgement cannot be questioned. Indeed, it is an essential attribute of a professional person that he or she is able to explain and, if need be, defend a judgement which has been made to the client, the client's family, and to elected representatives. In a democracy where authority to offer or withhold services is delegated by elected representatives to paid staff, that authority is underpinned by the particular skills and competence of the staff concerned.

The assessment of human needs cannot be considered in isolation from the particular resources available to meet them. Abstract statements about the need for warmth, food, shelter, and companionship must be translated by public agencies into terms that enable plans to be drawn up to respond to the deficiencies that occur. The organiser is concerned with the manner in which perceived needs can be met by the provision of a home help, but she will be aware of other needs of the client which, if unmet, will make it difficult or impossible for her own service to achieve its full potential. The process of assessment must, therefore, involve a broad appreciation of the client's situation as well as a recognition of the contribution that the home help service can make in meeting wider needs. Rarely, if ever, can an assessment of need for home help service be undertaken without some consultation with agencies or persons responsible for meeting other needs of the client.

AN APPROACH TO THE ASSESSMENT OF HUMAN NEEDS

Before examining the process of assessment in detail, it is necessary to consider the basic principles that surround this subject. An assessment carried out by a home help organiser is primarily an assessment of the person, his abilities, his expectations, and his aspirations; the organiser needs to know what tasks the client can perform, how long he has been incapacitated and the reason; she must know what help the client receives from those around him and the way he reacts to that help; she must ascertain how he views his current situation – whether he is stoically cheerful or depressed, critical of those around him or full of praise for their efforts on his behalf; she must form some judgement as to whether he can be expected to become more self-sufficient if he receives assistance or whether intervention by the service will confirm his sense of failure and defeat.

The assessment of the person is the key element in the home help assessment process. The approach and skills required are essentially the same as for any other assessment of social welfare need – whether it be for admission to an elderly persons' home, the provision of a day nursery place, structural alterations to enable a handicapped person to live at home, or the provision of a holiday for a handicapped child. The similarities in all these situations are that clients (or in the case of a child, his parents) require assistance from an official or semi-official agency in order to cope with personal, social, or emotional problems. The assessment must, therefore, start with the personalities of the people involved. The differences in the assessment process for the various types of need relate to the facts of the disability and the information needed to determine what services are required.

People usually have strong views about their own personal situation. They also have deep-seated reactions to being dependent on others – particularly statutory services. Clients who, superficially, appear to have the same needs, respond differently. One old person with a leg amputated will see this as a challenge to be overcome and may require little or no help, whereas another in similar circumstances will need encouragement and services to help him overcome his despair and depression so that he is prevented from withdrawing from life. Too often, assessment is seen as an examination of the rooms to be cleaned or the equipment available. Not only does such an approach ignore the central issue in any helping process – the client and his feelings – but it fails to build on any strength which may be present in the client and is likely to make him feel that he has been treated as less than human.

The core of any assessment of human abilities and potentiality is the personal interview, in which the client explains his circumstances and the interviewer uncovers the facts about the client's situation and, more importantly, how he sees them. Information derived from other sources, including that supplied by other organisations and by caring relatives and neighbours, plays a part in establishing for the organiser the background to the client's present situation, but it is during the personal interview with the client that his views can be ascertained about his problems and possible solutions to them.

It is sometimes difficult to establish which of the various people involved with a particular problem should be regarded as the client. For example, in a maternity case, is it the mother who is about to give birth or the father who is pacing the landing? In such circumstances the needs of both must be considered. It can be even more complex: with a confused and frail old person, the attitude of a caring neighbour may need to be taken into account just as much as the circumstances and wishes of the client. The organiser may sometimes weigh up the needs, wishes, and abilities of a large number of people concerned with the household to determine the best way of offering assistance. It is not uncommon to find that the most significant person is not the client but an anxious, perhaps overbearing, relative who has strong views about what is or is not required.

The assessment process itself can be a powerful form of intervention. The mere fact that the organiser formulates pertinent questions about the way in which the household functions, or could function, may prompt those involved to a new realisation of the extent of the problem or of ways of alleviating it. Relatives who say that an old or handicapped person cannot be left alone or cannot prepare his own meals may need to be asked to give reasons; in responding to the question they may come to a better understanding of the problem; indeed, they may begin to discern that the problem they are enunciating stems from their own anxiety, and that there is no reason why the client should not be left alone or prepare his own meals. By her implicit assumptions about human values which are communicated to the client, and by expressions of confidence in the capacity of the client to make decisions about his future, the organiser may be an important factor in achieving change. The discussion that the organiser promotes involving the client and those around him often continues well after she has completed her visit. Indeed, she may stimulate a dialogue between all the parties concerned that has never previously taken place.

The primary task of the organiser is to help the client and those caring for him to consider the problems, to contemplate the options for relieving them, and to weigh up the merits of these options. It is important that when the interview is ended the client feels he has reached his own decisions and that he regards the organiser as approachable in the event of the chosen option later being proved to be inappropriate. A simple maxim is that he who has the problem must find the solution. If the client or those providing care articulate a problem, the organiser's task is to help them plan how the problem can be overcome. The plan chosen may be the provision of a home help, but this is unlikely to solve the problem unless those concerned feel it to be appropriate.

By asking questions and guiding discussion an organiser can help the client and those caring for him to appreciate more fully the extent and nature of the problem. She may be able to disentangle complex issues that have led to misunderstandings and inappropriate responses in the past. For example, the organiser may learn that the client has declined an offer to attend a day centre because of a misunderstanding about transport arrangements or the cost; a mother may not appreciate that her mentally ill son is entitled to receive social security payments. The organiser can only draw out the full problems of the client and the household by encouraging a structured discussion of the total situation. To do this she must consciously strive to adopt an approach to interviewing which releases tension and stimulates an open discussion on issues that may be painful to those concerned; by doing so, she helps to release the potential of the client, the family, and the community to provide effective care. Yet this must be achieved within what is usually a very tight timescale for the organiser has many different duties to perform.

The organiser cannot discard her personality. She is as much a product of society as those she seeks to serve and will carry with her the prejudices and assumptions that are part of her individual make-up. Like the rest of us, she will constantly make judgements about human situations based on her own life experiences. A person whose task it is to assess the personal and emotional needs of others must have a stable personality and indefinable qualities generally known as judgement and integrity. Whilst it is not possible to make a good organiser out of someone who does not possess these qualities, they are not by themselves sufficient to ensure good or even satisfactory interviews and assessment. The organiser needs training in this area of her work, not as a means of informing her of techniques or to obtain a set of guidelines for use in interviewing, but to broaden her understanding of people and their needs, to make her aware of her own reaction to disability and human needs, and to help her become more consciously aware of how she can draw out and make use of the information and ideas she obtains during an interview. She will never be entirely satisfied with her performance; she will seek to modify her instinctive judgements by understanding how people behave under stress and how her personal intervention can help to build self-respect and a sense of dignity in others.

The training needs of organisers are discussed more fully in Chapter 12, but it may be helpful to indicate here some of the principles that underlie effective interviewing and assessment. A person who wishes to understand the social functioning of others must first and foremost be able to encourage people in need to express themselves and must recognise and respond to the individuality of the client regardless of his faults and failures. An organiser must come to terms with feelings of revulsion about women who neglect their children, husbands who beat their wives, and the mentally ill who may be demanding and aggressive. Whatever her thoughts as a private individual, when she acts in the role of home help organiser she is doing a professional job and she must not allow her personal likes and dislikes to intrude. Public services should be available to all citizens assessed according to their needs. They cannot be allocated on the grounds of personal prejudice or on concepts of moral worth left over from a bygone age. Judgements must be based on facts about needs, not on a sense of personal outrage or stifling sympathy.

In practice, if an organiser adopts a punitive or aggressive stance to clients who displease her or whose past behaviour is abhorrent to her, she will fail to carry out a meaningful assessment. Clients soon detect an unsympathetic listener and are reluctant to reveal problems that they believe will be greeted with disapproval. It is, therefore, important to demonstrate to the client that what he says is important and that he will not be criticised.

Many clients face the prospect of an interview with anxiety and sometimes anger. For them the interview may signify their sense of failure to manage their own affairs unaided. People who have been active and independent all their lives may resent growing infirmity. In such cases it is not uncommon for them to give vent to their frustration, anger, and hostility on the organiser. The organiser must be prepared for such eventualities and be ready to spend time discussing with the client his feelings about asking for help; he may need considerable reassurance that the organiser understands and respects his sense of personal outrage and loss of pride, and that he is valued as an individual. In this way the skilful interviewer diverts negative and aggressive feelings from a personal and damaging attack into a constructive discussion about dependency.

Another important principle, which must guide all those engaged in helping others, is that clients should be given as much responsibility as possible for decision-making about their own lives. Even clients who are so frail, confused, or socially incompetent that it would be manifestly wrong to expect them to make plans for their future, usually possess some residual understanding about what is happening to them. Time spent in explaining what is being planned, and why, is never wasted. This is also true for relatives and other caring persons who need to feel that their efforts at providing care are appreciated and their views taken into account. Sometimes a caring person has been carrying a heavy burden unaided; he or she may be pleased to be relieved of the burden of care, but may well feel offended if all her work is ignored by the organiser and alternative arrangements made with inadequate consultation.

Giving clients full opportunity to make decisions about their own future can be time-consuming. It is far easier and quicker (although less effective in the long run) to adopt an authoritarian approach telling the client and his relatives what to do and how and informing them what is to be arranged. Another approach that suits the personalities of some interviewers is over-protectiveness where the client is entreated to 'leave it all to me'. Either way the individuality of the client is not being recognised.

The organiser must never talk down to clients or relatives. Every aspect of the service should be discussed, so that the client sees the relevance of the service to his particular situation and feels that he is taking part in the decision about whether or not a home help will be provided, the number of hours required, and the work to be undertaken.

A principle common to all social welfare interviews is that of the confidentiality of information. The organiser represents the agency that employs her and the information she obtains belongs to her employers. She is not free to use it for other purposes, and the client is entitled to believe that any information imparted by him or on his behalf is used only for the purpose for which it was supplied.

In general, clients should know who is being asked to provide information for an assessment and should be given an opportunity to give assent or otherwise to the passing of that information. Similarly, clients have a right to feel secure that information supplied for a home help assessment will not be passed to a third person without consent; this includes relatives or other caring persons. Organisers must constantly use their discretion about sensitive information and must not assume that information imparted to them has already been passed to others. Wherever possible at least part of the assessment interview should be held in private with the client, to ensure that he is not inhibited in what he says by other people who may be present. Whether relatives should be seen separately from the client is a matter of judgement for the organiser. Certainly privacy sometimes enables relatives to give helpful information that would otherwise not come to light, but it can sometimes be an embarrassment for the organiser if she has information she cannot discuss with the client.

It is not possible to indicate precisely what information is required by an organiser to carry out a thorough assessment; this will vary considerably from case to case. What can be said with certainty, however, is that the organiser does not have the right to know everything about the individual and his life – only what is relevant to the assessment. There is no reason why the client should not be left with his secrets.

The confidentiality of information does not rest entirely with the organiser. It is important to ensure that information storage systems are secure. This has become increasingly important as social services records become computerised, and it is necessary to ensure that information placed on record by the organiser cannot be extracted by unauthorised persons. Clerks and typists who deal with confidential material on an everyday basis should be made aware of the importance attached to the privacy of records so that, for example, they do not give personal information on the telephone without being absolutely satisfied it is proper to do so. The swapping of idle chatter about the service and its clients should be discouraged. Not only is there a danger of names being overheard on buses or in restaurants, but in rural areas it may not be difficult for bystanders to know who is being discussed even though names are not mentioned; in any case, gossip in public places, even if not traceable to particular clients, is unlikely to impart a reassuring image of the service and those who work in it.

Elected representatives are entitled to have sufficient information to make policy decisions and to determine whether or not services are being provided in an appropriate manner. This has implications for the way in which confidential material is handled. A ratepayer who turns to a local councillor for help when a request for a home help is rejected may not expect full personal details to be relayed to the councillor. On the other hand, the councillor is entitled to have sufficient information to judge whether the refusal arose after careful consideration or was a callous and ill-thought-out act. The organiser's response will depend on the circumstances and the councillor's knowledge of the client. If in doubt the organiser should ask the client whether he objects to the councillor being informed of personal details. Similar principles apply to enquiries from Members of Parliament.

THE PROCESS OF ASSESSMENT

Assessment is composed of three basic elements: first, the gathering together of relevant information about the client and his problem; secondly, the assembling of the information that has been gathered so that the client's situation can be understood; and thirdly, the reviewing of options for action and deciding how the needs identified should be met. For convenience, these three elements are considered in sequence. In practice, they are interwoven in the assessment process: as the organiser assembles and reassembles the facts presented to her she seeks to understand the client's problem which, in turn, prompts her to ask for further information so that she can test out her beliefs about him and the nature of the problem. When she is ready to consider the courses of action open to her for meeting the client's needs, she may find it necessary to reappraise her understanding of the problem and to deal with those aspects of it she can most realistically tackle.

In that part of the process concerned with gathering information, the organiser is primarily concerned with establishing facts. What is the client's condition? What prevents him from functioning effectively? What aspects in his everyday life cause him the greatest difficulty? How does he cope with dressing, washing, cooking, feeding, cleaning, walking, shopping, and general household tasks? The answers to these questions require an act of judgement on the part of the organiser, for it is very seldom that the client's condition is static or that a simple 'yes' or 'no' will suffice. There may be disagreement among those who know the client best about how he manages his affairs. A general practitioner or health visitor may say he cannot prepare a meal, but this may be denied by the client or a relative. The organiser must attempt to establish a picture of how the client manages, accepting that her picture can never be entirely accurate in every detail.

Facts about people are seldom what they seem, and they are never straightforward. The client who says he cannot leave the house unaided may be telling the factual truth, but there may be no physical reason why he must remain at home – he may be depressed or lack the necessary confidence to go out. It is therefore important to establish the client's perception of his problem: how he feels about his domestic circumstances is just as much a fact to be taken into consideration as whether he can make his bed.

The most revealing part of an interview is not always what the client says but how he says it, what he looks like, and what he does. The client who avows that he can manage unaided but takes five minutes to cross the room obviously requires further investigation. Similarly, the organiser will carry her researches further if a client and his living room appear well cared for but the client says that he cannot manage and has no one to help him, for he may have high standards or be simply hiding his real concerns. The expectations and understanding of those around the client also represent important facts to be borne in mind. The over-protective neighbour who sees risks in everything the client does may be a significant factor in persuading him that he is incapacitated.

It is always important to enquire how the client has coped until now and what incident or incidents have made it necessary for help to be sought at this particular time. Sometimes the reason is easily understood: he has become unwell, or his wife has been admitted to hospital, leaving him alone and uncared for. It may then be possible to identify what support he was previously receiving and to see whether the home help service, either alone or in conjunction with others, can fill the gap.

With clients suffering from chronic or deteriorating conditions, the reasons why a request for help is made at a particular point in time can be very complex and it is essential for the organiser to gain as good an understanding as possible. This may require some persistence in questioning the client and those around him, including the referring agency. The service may be required because the family feel that the client has become so great a burden to them that they can no longer tolerate the work involved. This must be respected, but the perceptive organiser will wish to know which aspects of the burden represented the last straw. There may be ways of assisting short of replacing all the care which up to now has sustained the client in his own home. Matters may be brought to a head because the principal caring person wants a holiday, feels depressed, or is temporarily unwell; in such circumstances, the organiser may be able to arrange temporary help so that the previous form of care can be resumed in due course. Perhaps the carers wish to hand over responsibility because the client has begun to wander at night or has become incontinent, in which case the organiser will want to know whether medical advice has been sought, and whether other services, such as an incontinent laundry service or a night-sitter, could sufficiently relieve the burden.

Every client referred to a home help organiser is likely to be known to another social agency. Normally referrals are made by statutory or voluntary services which can supply basic background information about the client and his needs. The referring agency should always be asked why it is considered that the home help service is appropriate and what need it is thought should be met, for the expectations of other services are important factors to be taken into account. If after her investigation the organiser finds that her assessment is markedly different from that of the referring agency, she has a duty to communicate this and to see whether the differences in perception and understanding can be resolved.

The particular expertise of the referring agency must be recognised. The organiser is not omnicompetent; she must rely on the specialist knowledge and skills of others in forming judgements about the needs of clients and how they can be met. A social worker who has been working for several weeks with a client will have valuable information about how the household functions and the personal needs of those it contains. A medical officer, health visitor, or home nurse will have significant advice to give about a client's physical condition, his residual symptoms, and the likely course of an illness. These facts are highly relevant and must be taken into account during an assessment. The degree and type of help the organiser provides may depend in very large measure on medical advice. The organiser will certainly wish to know whether the client's disability is likely to be temporary or permanent or whether she should anticipate a steady deterioration. She will also need to be aware of the extent to which the client should be encouraged to engage in household and domestic duties as a means of rehabilitation.

In describing the facts that are required in order to form a realistic assessment of how the client can be helped, it has already been necessary to explain why they are required and how they can help the organiser to make her assessment. Each fact is a meaningless piece of information until it is compared with others to build up a picture of the client and his needs. Like a giant jigsaw, all the facts must be laid out in the organiser's mind so that the significant pieces can be identified, the inconsistencies examined and checked, and the overall pattern observed. The organiser needs to ask herself: What do these facts mean? What is it like to be this client? What is cause and what is effect? What can this client do for himself? What help is forthcoming from other caring persons? What aspect of the problem I have identified is one with which my particular service can assist? What aspects of the client's malfunctioning are beyond my competence or outside the scope of my service, and who should be responding to these needs?

The organiser will pose these questions to herself whilst she gathers information; as she builds up a mental picture of the client and his problem she will test out her assumptions and conjectures by formulating pertinent questions, or leading the discussion to an exploration of the issues that remain obscure to her. But there is no reason why her ruminations about what, why, how, and when should remain a private reverie, for if they help her to understand the client's situation they will surely also be of assistance to the client himself and to others who are involved with him. In any case, if the client is to understand why he is to receive a service and what it is meant to achieve, he needs to know what is in the mind of the organiser. It is therefore often helpful for the organiser to summarise the situation with the client, giving him an opportunity to agree or dispute what is said. If, at the end of this stage, all the parties have reached agreement about the nature of the problem to be solved, there is a greater chance of the service that is eventually provided meeting real needs. Similarly, in the event of it being decided that the home help service is not required, the client will have the satisfaction of knowing that the decision was taken with a full understanding of all the issues.

Having collected the relevant facts and considered their meaning, the organiser is then ready to draw together all the strands and make her assessment of the problem. The word *assessment* is preferred to the medical expression *diagnosis* because it more accurately reflects the process involved. *Diagnosis* implies a set of ready-made labels which can be affixed to the client's record classifying him as senile, frail, or incontinent, rather like a doctor might indicate a patient as suffering from whooping cough, measles, or diphtheria; it signifies differences in quality between one state and another. *Assessment*, on the other hand, conveys the concept of measurement or an evaluation of a series of factors each of which may vary in importance.

The organiser should share her conclusions with the client and review with him the possible options that occur to her. The service can only be provided if the client meets the criteria of need approved by the social services committee or established by senior managers. The organiser should avoid the temptation to provide a service simply because the client is distressed or in obvious difficulty. She has a responsibility to make the best use of the resources at her disposal and this means that her judgements must be carefully thought out. If the client does not need a home help or would be better served by another agency she must say so and, if need be, assist him to locate a more appropriate source of help. In determining the best course of action the organiser must bear in mind the twin aims of the service – to find solutions to problems of functioning and to promote capacities for growth within clients.

There can be no single formula for meeting individual need. The client will require a widely different input from the home help depending on whether the object of the service is to provide care or rehabilitation and depending on the different household circumstances that prevail. The organiser should always make a written note of her assessment and the principal factors surrounding the decision to provide or not to provide a service. This is not only a protection in the event of a query at a later date: it enables the organiser to compare her findings in subsequent assessment interviews with the same client and to identify the changes that may have occurred. Proper recording is also an aid to learning.

The assessment of need is not fully completed when the organiser has formulated a plan based on the circumstances of the client. She must next weigh the needs identified against the needs of other clients known to her, so that she can determine the priority to be offered to that particular client. The priority rating could depend on the degree of need, the availability of alternative means of assistance (for example, relatives and neighbours), as well as a comparison of the client's need with that of others. Not all clients with a demonstrable need for the service can be assisted, and it is the responsibility of the employing authority to ensure that guidelines are laid down to assist and protect the organiser who is obliged to refuse an application, or withdraw a service prematurely, in order to offer help to a client whose needs are considered to be greater.

The home help selected for the client should, if possible, be chosen not at random but on the basis of the qualities she is known to possess. Home helps vary in their capacities to work with different kinds of clients. Some are good with the elderly but others soon strike up warm relationships with children. Some achieve miracles with soap and water whereas others have aptitudes for working alongside clients and encouraging them to greater efforts at independence. Careful matching of home help and client can help to ensure job satisfaction for the home help; since, in many instances, she spends more time with the client than any other person, it is important that the client is able to develop a personal liking for her.

Restraints imposed by distance may cause problems in the provision of a service in rural areas; and sometimes special requirements for extended hours, early morning working, or the need for residential provision may make it difficult or impossible for an organiser to meet the needs she identifies. It is important that the organiser sees her home helps as a total resource and that she endeavours to provide the best possible service bearing in mind their different abilities and availability. Beyond that, she requires a management structure that enables her to draw upon the resources of other districts and areas when she is unable to meet pressing needs from within her existing provision. Only in this way can the service of the authority as a whole be used effectively.

In discussing a new client with a home help, the organiser will draw attention to the tasks to be undertaken, specify special needs, and indicate the extent to which the client may be helped to undertake tasks for himself. If it is known that the client's condition may deteriorate, the home help should be alerted to the kind of symptoms that could develop.

It is also helpful if she is told of the approximate length of time that the service will be provided. She will need to know about the assistance being offered by relatives and neighbours, the general circumstances of the accommodation, and the state of appliances such as vacuum cleaners, together with a special note of any hazards to health and safety that may be apparent.

In particularly complex situations in which it is proposed that the home help should monitor changes in the household to assist other professionals to assess progress – i.e. in respect of child abuse or acute mental illness – it is desirable for the organiser to issue a written statement to the home help detailing the duties to be undertaken and the items to be reported.

The human condition is constantly changing. The provision of a home help will have an impact on the client and the way he responds to problems, while external influences such as medical treatment and the availability of family and friends to offer help may conspire to render the original assessment out of date. It is important that the circumstances of clients are kept under regular review and that adjustments in provision are made in the light of experience. The needs of some can be expected to change rapidly whilst others are likely to remain constant for long periods; the intervals between reviews should be varied to suit individual circumstances.

The assessment and review of need is at the centre of the home help organiser's professional task. She must create a balance between the wishes of the client (or those representing him), assessed needs, and the resources available. Sometimes the wishes expressed by the client or his family are unrealistic and cannot be met, because the need is not established or because there are insufficient resources at the disposal of the organiser; on other occasions it may be necessary to persuade a reluctant client to accept help. In exercising her judgement and skill the organiser must always try to reconcile wishes, needs, and resources in a way that the client finds broadly acceptable or at least understandable; failure to do so will lead to dissatisfaction and the possibility of subsequent friction between the client and home help.

In reviewing the needs of an existing client the organiser can be greatly assisted by the knowledge and experience of the home help. She is an invaluable source of information about the client's capacity to undertake tasks unaided, and of the willingness and ability of other members of the household or neighbourhood to provide assistance. The dialogue between organiser and home help is an essential ingredient of assessment reviews, and it is important that home helps are introduced to some of the concepts of assessment in their training, so that they can take a full and continuous part in this aspect of the service. An organiser who has insufficient time to discuss clients and their needs with her home helps is denied the opportunity of benefiting from their knowledge when reviewing clients, but is also unable to test the validity of her assessments against the subsequent experience of her staff.

A study in Cumbria (Gwynne and Fean 1978) revealed a considerable discrepancy between the service provided by home helps and the intentions of the organisers. This may arise because of inaccurate assessments or because home helps are not properly briefed; also, needs change over time and home helps respond naturally to changing situations which they may not report. It is likely that some home helps, because of the extent of their experience and their proximity to clients, are better at assessing needs than some organisers, although it is equally true that some are not and that the service suffers through an absence of adequate supervision. Unfortunately, regular reviews of client need and case discussions between home helps and organisers are among the first duties to suffer when caseloads rise and staff find themselves working under pressure.

Organisers require accurate information about the condition of each client because it is frequently necessary to redeploy a home help from an existing client to meet urgent priority needs elsewhere; without a thorough knowledge of clients currently being helped the organiser is unable to make realistic judgements. Poor assessments by organisers soon lead to frustration by clients and home helps alike. Organisers should have a clear idea of the unmet needs in their areas; only in this way can they ensure that senior managers and elected representatives are able to be informed of shortfalls in provision and the need for new developments.

The termination of the service or a reduction in the number of hours provided should be carefully planned. Abrupt changes, even if accompanied by explanations, can be seen by clients as personal rejection. Even emotionally stable clients may respond with anger and resentment if suddenly told that the service they have come to rely upon is to be discontinued. Where, on assessment, it is thought likely that the service will be withdrawn at a later date, this should be explained, so that changes come as no surprise and any other necessary arrangements can be made in good time.

Whatever skills and experience are brought to bear by managers in the service and the home helps they employ, there will, from time to time, be mistakes, failures in communication, and dissatisfied clients. The assessment of need is not an exact science and, in any case, circumstances can change to render an assessment inappropriate. The number of complaints about the service is remarkably low, but when problems arise they are seldom brought about by the callous or indifferent behaviour of a member of staff. Indeed, it is more usual for a situation to be mishandled through the sheer anxiety of staff to do the best they possibly can for the client. As Franklin D. Roosevelt might have said, 'The main thing that organisers need to be anxious about is anxiety itself'.

Staff who are recruited and trained to serve the public have a strong desire to do their job well and to help members of the public with their problems. When circumstances conspire to make this difficult or impossible, considerable personal anxiety can be aroused within the helper which may lead her to make inappropriate decisions. The frustration and sense of personal failure provoked by being unable to respond to the needs of others can be a considerable burden, particularly if the client directs indignation and anger at the interviewer. This must be recognised by managers at all levels in the service so that when mistakes occur they can be handled with understanding and staff can learn from them.

There are a number of ways in which interviewers in all public services deal with their own anxieties and attempt to avoid or reduce the personal tension and guilt feelings that are created when they are confronted by problems they cannot solve. One defence mechanism commonly used is to pass the client on to another service without first verifying that such a referral is appropriate. It is still quite common for clients to be sent from one public agency to another in the mistaken hope that the next person will find a solution to the problem. It is important that managers in the home help service make good use of the expertise to be found in other services, but to do so they must ensure that a referral is appropriate and not used as a means of reducing their own anxiety when they are forced to turn away a client.

A variant of this problem is when the interviewer defends herself by telling the client or his relatives that some other agency is responsible for the problem. 'Of course, your mother should be in hospital' or 'This house is unsuitable; the housing department should rehouse you' are neat phrases that absolve the home help service of any responsibility for the privations and unpleasantness of a difficult situation. Such statements may ease tension in the interviewer, but do so at the expense of building up stress in the client or his family. In certain circumstances such statements may be true, but the organiser is claiming an expertise she does not possess if she presumes to announce who should or should not be in hospital or be rehoused.

Organisers are only too well aware of the problems that face them when clients declare 'The doctor said I must have a home help' or 'The health visitor said you were wrong to reduce the number of hours'. Some clients, of course, attempt to substantiate their eligibility for help by using the name of their doctor, health visitor, or another person held in high esteem, so it should not always be assumed that statements alleged to have been made by staff in other agencies are true.

One trap that clerks and inexperienced organisers sometimes fall into is to promise more than the service can deliver. A telephone call seeking urgent assistance for a client in distress is a signal for anyone employed in the home help service to respond, unthinkingly, 'Yes, of course, we'll send someone at once'. If the promise can be kept and immediate assistance provided the service will earn another increment of gratitude and respect and all will be well, but the clerk or organiser must be realistic; it is tempting to respond to urgent and emotional appeals for assistance by making promises that cannot be fulfilled. It can be difficult to say no, and even more difficult to respond helpfully to an angry and harassed client who asks in desperation, 'What can I do?' There is little satisfaction in declining to help people in need, but there are practical limitations to the service that can be provided and it is better to be realistic than to raise false hopes. The home help service is not the custodian of the nation's conscience and cannot be expected to solve all society's problems.

9 · Charging policies

In a modern complex society the State provides a wide range of services to meet social and personal need. However, the extent of such services and the degree to which the cost falls on those who use them vary greatly between countries and between different parts of the same country. For practical reasons some public services must be funded communally, because there is no sensible way of establishing the cost of the provision for individual persons or households. Thus the cost of the police, of defence, the fire service, street lighting, the maintenance of highways, and many other services must be raised by way of public rates and taxes. Other services such as education, health, housing, and social welfare can be related to specific individuals or households, and it is a matter of political judgement whether it is reasonable, practical, or desirable to levy a charge on the user and, if so, whether all users should pay the full cost or be subject to an assessment of means. Different countries have reached different solutions to the question of operating and funding personal services; some services that are regarded as essential public provision in one country, and are heavily subsidised, are left entirely to private provision in another.

The legal framework within which public authorities charge for services, and the various practices adopted, defy rational explanation or logic; their roots lie in history and tradition and have been moulded by political judgements over time. Public services have grown up piecemeal. Most sprang from the enterprise of voluntary organisations and became part of statutory provision when there was a public awareness and acceptance of their value. The fragmented origins of the various strands now comprising the personal social services are an important fact;

different services were developed at different times to meet different needs. Many of the inconsistencies and anomalies that accompany current charging policies have existed for a long time. Indeed, the following statement from the Minority Report of the Royal Commission on the Poor Laws, which reported in 1909, remains true three-quarters of a century after it was written.

'Practically all Local Authorities affording Public Assistance in any form . . . have the power, in respect of some of their services, to charge the whole or part of the cost upon the individual benefited. . . . These powers differ from service to service and from Authority to Authority, alike in the amount or proportion of the expense that is chargeable; in the discretion allowed to the Authority to charge or not to charge as it sees fit; in the conditions attached to the charge or exemption from payment; in the degree of poverty entitling to exemption. . . . This chaotic agglomeration of legal powers, conferred on different Authorities at different dates, for different purposes, . . . proceed upon no common principle.'

Views vary about the extent to which the cost of public services should be met by the user, views which are often based on confused and conflicting opinions about the purpose and effect of charges. Roy Parker (1980 : 24) has identified five main purposes for levying charges in respect of personal services. They are:

(1) to raise revenue;
(2) to reduce demand;
(3) to check extravagant use;
(4) to shift the pattern of care by making particular services more or less attractive;
(5) for symbolic purposes, i.e. to make controversial proposals more acceptable or to demonstrate cost consciousness.

The degree to which charges succeed in achieving these objectives is open to debate.

A sixth purpose for the existence of charges is sometimes advanced – that public services are likely to be more sensitive and responsive to the needs and wishes of consumers if clients make a direct financial contribution towards their cost. Those who support this philosophy point to the fact that in the commercial world consumers relate their satisfaction to the cost of their purchases in order to decide whether or not they have made a good buy; their pattern of consumption then determines the quantity, quality, and the type of service offered to the public. Where services are paid for by rates and taxes the normal market forces by which consumers influence supply are not applicable but are replaced by political judgements. This can mean that decisions do not correspond to the wishes of consumers, who have few opportunities to indicate personal preferences or influence the future pattern of supply. It is difficult to conceive of a system that could be developed in the United Kingdom in the foreseeable future which would give significant numbers of consumers the ability to meet the cost of the service they require; it is, therefore, important to develop other means by which consumer reaction and preferences can be identified and used to influence provision.

In some localities it can be shown that the costs of making financial assessments on clients, sending accounts, and collecting charges outweigh the resultant income, while in others the income derived from making charges represents a significant contribution towards meeting the cost of the service. This is a field of activity where ideals, principles, and practical considerations must be weighed in the balance and compromises sought.

Statutes decree that some public services must be provided free whilst others must be accompanied by a charge; local authorities are empowered to determine whether or not to make a charge in respect of certain services. The fact that many health and education services are free whilst social services authorities are empowered, and sometimes required, to charge for services meeting similar needs creates serious anomalies, as the following table shows.

There is no logic in a law which provides for accommodation in respect

Table 7 *Charging for services*

type of service	health service provision (free)	education provision (free)	social services provision (chargeable)
residential care of the elderly	hospital	—	elderly persons' home
domiciliary care of the elderly	community nurse and health visitor	—	home help
children's residential services	hospital	boarding school	community home
children's day care	hospital	school/nursery class	day nursery
day care of the physically and mentally handicapped	hospital	—	day unit

of a child or elderly person in hospital free of charge yet insists on a charge for local authority residential care. There is a widespread belief that medical care and education are intrinsically desirable activities and that social class or income should not be a barrier to their use, whereas the reception of children or old people into residential care, because their families can no longer meet their needs, is somehow less deserving, and is therefore accompanied by a financial penalty. The fact that persons requiring care for medical or educational purposes are placed in one category and those requiring care on social welfare grounds are placed in another, and that these two categories have remained fairly constant since at least the end of the second world war, suggests that they are in accordance with what the community believes to be broadly right.

Charging policies in relation to domiciliary services can be seen to relate generally to their institutional counterpart. Home nursing and home teaching services are free and relate to hospital care and schooling which are also free. The home help service is chargeable and relates to residential services for children and old people which are also chargeable. Even if some form of logic can be found that explains why services relating to medicine and education are free whilst those concerned with social welfare are chargeable, it must be acknowledged that services cannot always be neatly classified under these headings. The home help service promotes health as well as social welfare; it prevents the need for hospital care as well as the need for local authority residential services. Thus an elderly or handicapped person who refuses to accept a home help because of the cost may be placed at risk of requiring admission to hospital, which is free to him but infinitely more expensive for the community.

The law permits considerable flexibility to a social services authority as to the extent to which it will charge for services, except that charges must be made in respect of the residential care of children, the elderly, and handicapped adults – handicapped children can be accommodated free of charge. However, the law creates a distinction between services for which charges must have regard to the means of the client and those for which charges can be levied irrespective of means. Under Schedule 8 of the National Health Service Act of 1977, any charge made for the home help service in England and Wales must have regard to the means of the client.

Adults and children in the United Kingdom who are severely disabled, physically or mentally, and who require considerable care from those around them, are entitled to a weekly tax-free attendance allowance. A person caring for someone in receipt of an attendance allowance may, in some circumstances, be entitled to an invalid care allowance. As these allowances have been introduced to enable the disabled and their families to make their own care arrangements, it may be argued that recipients should contribute financially towards the cost of home help provision; yet those authorities that provide a free service do not recoup income from that source.

Thus two doctrines of social welfare, each valid in itself, when combined create unfairness and confusion. The notion that the disadvantaged are entitled to sufficient income to exercise choice in how they meet their needs receives widespread support; so does the notion that social welfare services should be provided as of right and at no cost to the needy. When both doctrines are applied together it is possible for clients to have their cake and eat it but, as yet, it must be admitted the cake is not particularly fruity.

SOME GENERAL CONSIDERATIONS

A bewildering range of charging policies prevails for the home help service, and in recent years a number of authorities have changed their approach to recover a larger proportion of their costs or to produce a charging system which is thought to be fairer for their localities. In such a complex area fairness is in the eye of the beholder, and even those authorities that have unashamedly revised their procedures in order to raise more income can argue that only by so doing can they maintain or increase the level of service. Fairness between different clients and client groups must be balanced by fairness to the ratepayers generally and to potential clients, whose expectations of receiving a service may be diminished unless income from charges can be ploughed back into the service.

Three distinct approaches to charging can be identified. They may be operated singly, or combined in a variety of ways to produce different levels of income and to gather that income from different groups in terms of type of disability, age, extent of service received, or ability to pay. The three methods are:

(1) a free service to every client;
(2) financial assessment of clients so that each pays according to his means and the extent of the service allocated;
(3) a flat rate charge to each client irrespective of his means and the extent of the service provided.

The principal variations and combinations of these systems are listed below:

(1) a free service to all clients;
(2) a free service to certain client groups;

(3) financial assessment of all clients with a minimum charge;
(4) financial assessment of clients with a nil assessment for those on supplementary benefit;
(5) financial assessment of clients with a nil assessment for those with incomes at supplementary benefit level;
(6) financial assessment with a maximum weekly charge;
(7) a standard flat rate charge for all clients irrespective of the extent of the service provided;
(8) a flat rate charge for all clients, with certain exceptions such as those on supplementary benefit or over a certain age;
(9) a flat rate charge with a financial assessment for those on higher incomes.

Further variations arise between authorities from the level of minimum, maximum, and flat rate charges adopted, as well as in the generosity or otherwise of the regulations relating to income and capital for assessment purposes.

Authorities that have adopted assessment procedures frequently assess large numbers of clients to pay nothing. However, a number of authorities in the United Kingdom have abolished charges altogether for the home help service; this policy has been much acclaimed by staff working in the service and the Institute of Home Help Organisers has pressed for its universal application.

The development of a free service began soon after the creation of social services departments in 1971. By the following year four local authorities in England were offering a free service, and by 1975 the number had increased to eleven; in 1978 it was at least fifteen, including two English counties, seven London boroughs and six metropolitan districts. The Northern Ireland Central Personal Social Services Advisory Committee reported in 1978 that 'The cost of a free home help service would not, in our opinion, be excessive when set against the present high administrative costs of assessing and collecting recipients' contributions and the fact that a high proportion of the service is already provided free of charge' (1978 : 35). However, in 1980 the Northern Ireland Department of Health and Social Services did 'not consider it opportune at present to introduce a completely free service' but decided that it should be free for those aged 75 and over and those in receipt of supplementary benefit or family income supplement (Circular 1/80).

The London Borough of Hackney, one of the first authorities in the country to abolish charges for the home help service, found in 1972 that 93 per cent of clients had a nil assessment, that 2 per cent met the full charge, and the remainder were assessed to pay part of the charge; taking into account the cost of assessment and collection there would be an overall saving by switching to a free service. However, such figures must be interpreted with caution. The assessment scale adopted by Hackney was more generous than most: the authority was recovering 1 per cent of gross costs against the then national average of 10 per cent, although average household incomes in the borough were no doubt lower than in most authorities. Had Hackney's assessment scales conformed more closely to the national average, income would have been higher and the decision to introduce a free service might have been more difficult. All that can be said with certainty is that the ratio of costs to revenue is much higher with assessments than, for example, flat rate charges, while of course free services have no collection costs.

Arguments in favour of levying charges relate to political and economic considerations. There are no professional arguments for retaining charges. The task of staff is to assess the needs of the individual and provide the appropriate service for the number of hours required. This process becomes clouded when clients are concerned about the cost and decide to restrict their use of the service because of the charge. It is frustrating for organisers to know that clients in need are denied a service and that provision is rationed, not by a system of priorities, but by ability or willingness to pay. Whilst charges may dampen demand they do not affect the extent of need – merely the level at which demand is made vocal.

It is likely that free services lead to an increase in demand; certainly the skills of organisers to judge the extent of need and to weigh priorities between different clients for the use of scarce resources are placed under extreme pressure, but the professional assessment of need is the first and foremost function of managers in the service. The slow development of free provision in the 1970s marked a watershed for the service: it signified an acceptance that home help organisers had achieved a professional status, and that their skilful judgement about need could stand as the only criterion for allocating substantial local authority resources.

It has long been recognised that the benefits of the home help service are such that certain clients who do not request the service should be persuaded to accept it. In such cases it is hardly reasonable to expect them to pay. It is, therefore, customary in most authorities for an organiser or other senior manager to have power to remit charges in individual cases, and in some authorities specific categories of client are exempted from payment, for example, long-term users or disorganised families in which the home help performs a rehabilitative or educative role.

A number of authorities have introduced specialist home care services to provide extended cover which keeps people out of hospital or enables them to return home from hospital earlier than would otherwise be possible. Such services are often provided free of charge for a limited period; in Avon the service of a home aide is free for six weeks following hospital discharge; in Birmingham fifteen hours can be free; and in the London Borough of Kensington and Chelsea a free service is provided for up to four weeks after hospital discharge.

The declining proportion of maternity cases and the rising numbers of the elderly in the workload have led to a gradual decline in the proportion of total costs met by charges. Between 1959/60 and 1978/79 the proportion of costs recovered in England fell from about 12 per cent to 4.7 per cent. Since then the growing popularity of flat rate charges by local authorities has almost certainly raised the proportion of costs recovered. There is a wide variation. In 1978/79 the county recovering the highest proportion of costs was Northamptonshire at 18.7 per cent; the highest metropolitan district was Sefton at 9.3 per cent.

Some arguments advanced for a free service are of dubious validity. For example, it is sometimes said that clients meeting the full cost can be very demanding and treat their home helps like servants, or that it is difficult to withdraw a service from someone willing and able to pay the full charge. These statements are undeniably true, but it would be wrong to make the service free merely to retain more control over clients. Users of public services have precious few opportunities to influence the quality and quantity of provision. Organisers and home helps must find ways of dealing with manipulative clients, ways based on a knowledge of human relationships and a skill in dealing with people who are depressed, angry, sick, or eccentric.

No authority in the United Kingdom expects all clients to meet the full economic cost of the service, but approaches vary considerably between authorities to the extent that probably no two areas have adopted precisely the same criteria for levying charges. The method of charging adopted by an authority, the percentage of costs recovered, and the incidence of charges on clients with different incomes, reflect the political views of the particular local authority.

It is clear that however sensitive charging policies are made, and however skilfully they are applied, some clients will find the process distasteful; moreover, some who have real needs that should be met will not be prepared to take full advantage of the service, and as a result the quality of their lives will suffer to the extent that, in some instances, other and more expensive forms of intervention by public services will be required. The price of this rejection was £7 million in 1978/79 – less the cost of collection.

Audrey Hunt's survey (1970 : 19) found that over 71 per cent of elderly clients paid nothing. The National Council of Home Help Services calculated that in 1975 over 80 per cent of clients in Great Britain were receiving a free service (1975 : 8). Maternity cases are probably the only client group where a large proportion are meeting a significant part of the cost. The debate about charging policies and the morality or otherwise of levying charges must be seen against this background.

The wide acceptance of the principle that it is reasonable to levy charges for the home help service raises questions of whether and how such charges should be levied on persons whose sole income is derived from supplementary benefits. There are two distinct ways of looking at this problem, which has led to considerable conflict over the years between social security agencies – the National Assistance Board, the Supplementary Benefits Commission, and the Department of Health and Social Security – and local authorities.

The local authority argument, simply put, is that it is the role of central government to provide an adequate income maintenance system and that the system should enable recipients to make reasonable payments for necessary services. In 1951 the two major local authority associations argued that much local authority expenditure was met from government grant, and that it could not have been the intention of Parliament that this money would be spent by local authorities 'to relieve the National Assistance Board of their financial responsibility for the relief of poverty' (*Joint Memorandum* 1951).

The response from the National Assistance Board was that persons in receipt of national assistance should be treated no differently from other people with similar incomes, and that there would be no overall saving of public expenditure if home help charges for people on national assistance were met by the board. But this did not entirely satisfy local authorities since about two-thirds of home help clients were in receipt of national assistance; they felt it was unfair that they should be required to provide a costly service to such a large number of clients who, because of the levels of allowances set by central government, could pay little or nothing towards the cost.

A circular issued in 1965 by the Ministry of Health urged local authorities not to charge recipients on national assistance or those whose incomes were at a similar level (Circular 25/65 : para. 12). It revealed that more than half of local authorities levied charges on clients in receipt of national assistance. The National Assistance Board and its successor, the Supplementary Benefits Commission, were prepared to make a contribution towards the cost of charges levied on their claimants, but made it clear that they found the additional work burdensome. In Scotland authorities were prohibited from charging supplementary benefit claimants.

By 1980 expenditure cuts imposed on local authorities were causing them to examine carefully all areas of income, to see whether more could be raised to enable them to preserve the level of services or avoid cuts of an extreme nature. Many authorities reviewed their system of home help charges and for the first time extended them to supplementary benefit claimants. To justify their actions, local authorities declared that it was the responsibility of government to pay adequate incomes to the poor and needy. The Supplementary Benefits Commission paid steadily increasing sums in respect of home help provision: in 1977 it was reported that 18,000 recipients of supplementary benefit received regular additional payment from the commission to cover home help charges; by 1979 the number had risen to 24,000. In an uncharacteristically blunt statement the Supplementary Benefits Commission declared in 1980 that 'Any authority making charges for this service to people – usually elderly and frail – so poor that they live on supplementary benefit, ought to be ashamed of itself'.

The government was asking for cuts in public expenditure; it could see no advantage in transferring costs from local authorities to the supplementary benefit system. The opportunity was therefore taken in the 1980 Social Security Act, and the regulations that accompanied it, to preclude additions to supplementary benefit in respect of local authority home help charges, although payments could still be made in respect of privately arranged domestic help. The long-standing dispute between local and central government about who should meet the cost of home help services to the poorest sections of society was therefore resolved in favour of the government. But some authorities continued to levy charges on supplementary benefit claimants.

CHARGING SYSTEMS

Although administratively complex, the assessment of each client's ability to pay on a sliding scale according to income and the extent of service received is undoubtedly the fairest way of levying charges. It is also the method most commonly adopted by United Kingdom local authorities. Criticisms of this system are generally based on the administrative costs involved, the adverse reaction of clients to means testing, and the tendency for home help organisers and their clerks to be overburdened with administrative and financial detail at the expense of activities more likely to benefit clients.

Whatever method is used to recover costs from clients it is bound to be unpopular and deter some clients in need from applying for service, but means tests have a particular odium of their own. The fact that so many statutory benefits and services are provided subject to a means test, despite the almost universal distaste for them, suggests that the advantages in terms of income and equity cannot readily be found in any other system. However skilfully information is sought on which to make an assessment some people feel humiliated by the process, which emphasises their low economic and social status. Some decline to answer questions about their income and outgoings, preferring to forgo the service altogether or to pay the full charge. There is sometimes a feeling of resentment among the elderly who have saved for their old age, only to find that they are assessed to pay a higher charge arising from the savings they have accumulated. Because of the complexity of the assessment process and the need to verify figures supplied, recipients do not always know the charge until after the service has commenced; this is unsatisfactory. The impact of multiple means testing produces unintended results with a marginal increase in income leading to a reduction in net income; the complexities are such that few people can detect the effect and the extent of the problem is therefore unknown.

Many home help organisers and clerks have expressed their dissatisfaction at being required to make financial assessments. Such work takes them away from what they see as their primary task, of establishing and meeting social need, to processing time sheets and preparing information for accounts. Furthermore, they find it unpleasant to pry into the personal affairs of frail and handicapped clients whose memories may be faulty and who may have only vague ideas of the amount and source of their income or the extent of their capital assets. It is sometimes necessary for organisers to look through personal belongings of handicapped clients to discover bank books, rent cards, and other documents; this they find unpleasant. Where home help staff are responsible for pursuing bad debts the conflict of role as well as the time involved can cause serious problems.

There is general agreement that some clients and potential clients are deterred by charges and that the higher the charge the more likely clients are to refuse service. Evidence on these points arises from almost every study that seeks the views of clients, home helps, and organisers.

Amelia Harris found that some clients preferred to pay the full charge rather than reveal their income to the home help organiser (1968 : 19); one such client said she paid the charge direct to the home help and would not want her to know of her depressed financial circumstances. Amelia Harris also thought some people in need did not apply for a home help because of the charge, although it was not known whether all such people were aware of the true cost. Audrey Hunt confirmed these findings (1970 : 343). The majority of the fifty-four home help organisers she interviewed believed that some people were put off applying for a home help or gave up having one because of the charge; the elderly were most frequently mentioned, followed by maternity cases. Similarly, the majority of organisers who knew clients who had discontinued using the service because of the charge thought there had been hardship as a result. Mrs Hunt also learned that clients who received a service for more than two hours a week were more likely to receive it free than those who had less time allocated; she concluded that one explanation might be that those who were required to pay for their home help restricted the numbers of hours to match what they felt they could afford.

A review of home help services in England by the Department of Health and Social Security which covered 141 local authorities quoted a number of organisers as saying that whenever charges were increased there was a notable reduction in requests for help, and that some clients asked for the service to be supplied for fewer hours (DHSS 1973 : 31). This study also drew attention to the fact that employers sometimes became irritated by repeated requests to confirm earnings where long-term help was being provided.

It is, of course, important that information supplied by clients about their income and expenditure is correctly recorded so that accurate assessments can be made. It is possible to verify earnings and other regular income by checking documentation or by writing to employers or pension funds, but it is impossible to know whether all capital assets have been declared. Trust plays a very important part in making an assessment. The nature and extent of income can change dramatically and so it is necessary to reassess clients on a regular basis: twice a year is probably adequate for many clients, with at most an annual check on those receiving supplementary benefit.

A typical assessment scheme requires the organiser to list all sources of income and then to deduct certain outgoings to arrive at net disposable income. Sometimes certain items of income are disregarded – such as boarding-out allowances paid for foster children. Capital may be dealt with by taking into account interest received or by assuming a notional income according to the extent of the assets. The deductions are usually rent and rates and other necessary expenses such as fares to work and insurance, together with an allowance for each adult or child. The National Council of Home Help Services found in 1975 that most authorities related these deductions to the supplementary benefit scale of allowances, although many were more generous (1975 : 11). A percentage or a fixed sum may then be deducted from the net disposable income to arrive at the net assessable income, and the resultant figure can then be compared with a sliding scale of charges to determine the amount the client must pay. This scale may be constant or it may be weighted to place a greater or lesser burden on clients at either end of the scale. The scale may be related to the weekly payment or to the hourly charge; in the latter case, which is more common, the cost to the client is determined by the hourly charge set against the number of hours allocated.

A maximum or standard hourly charge is normally fixed, beyond which clients are not expected to pay irrespective of their means; this charge is usually derived from the average hourly cost of the service, but the figure may be arrived at by adding in all or part of the administrative overheads. Where this is done the maximum charge is likely to exceed greatly the cost of privately arranged domestic help, and this may have an impact on demand. Audrey Hunt (1970 : 341) found that thirteen areas out of fifty-four had established maximum hourly charges that were less than the pay of home helps, so that even clients charged at the maximum were subsidised. The National Council of Home Help Services (1975 : 18) found that maximum hourly charges varied enormously across the country with, for example, the average figure in Welsh counties being 2.5 times higher than in Scottish regions; English counties were 17 per cent higher than metropolitan districts.

The sheer volume of work in assessing all home help clients makes it desirable to find rule-of-thumb methods that exclude large numbers of clients from the assessment process. This can be achieved by adopting a policy of making no charge to recipients of supplementary benefit, as in most areas this excludes about two-thirds of all clients. Where services to supplementary benefit claimants are free it is equitable to ensure that clients on similar levels of income also receive the service free, but the National Council of Home Help Services study quoted above (1975 : 20) revealed that a number of authorities providing service free to those on supplementary benefit charged other clients on low incomes.

An assessment system can be modified by combining it with a minimum charge, thus ensuring that every recipient makes a contribution towards the cost, although this does not meet with the approval of the Department of Health and Social Security since it levies a charge on supplementary benefit claimants. This combination can produce considerably more income than assessment alone. An assessment system together with a nil assessment for those at supplementary benefit level generally leads to lower administrative costs.

Charging policies and professional direction can be in conflict. A decision to provide an intensive service to clients who are most vulnerable, rather than to offer a small number of hours to a great many, may not be achievable if charging policies lead the clients concerned to decline the service. This could face staff and committee members with the embarrassment of explaining and defending an underspent budget when needy clients, within the agreed criteria of eligibility, are not assisted. Clients who need intensive help may deteriorate without it and require expensive and inappropriate admission to hospital or an elderly persons' home. The most needy can be encouraged to meet the cost if the authority adopts a maximum weekly charge so that however many hours of service are provided the client pays for only the first three or four. Similar results can be achieved by restricting the weekly charge to a fixed percentage of net disposable income. Assessment can also be combined with the provision of free services to certain client groups – for example, those over 75 years in Northern Ireland.

It is necessary for authorities operating assessment schemes to review the scale of charges on a regular basis in order to take account of inflation, both in terms of the cost of providing the service and because of the general rise in money incomes for clients. Financial procedures in some authorities dictate that unless charges are increased to match inflation the social services committee budget will not be increased to meet the shortfall; thus a decision not to raise charges may require a corresponding reduction in the home help or other services controlled by the social services committee. Most authorities review charges on an annual basis when social security payments are raised or when home help wages increase.

A charging system that overcomes most of the objections to means testing is the flat rate charge to all clients. This enables each client to be told at the outset the exact amount of his contribution, it avoids the need to collect information about income and expenditure from individual clients, it frees organisers from anxieties about whether particular clients will be willing to pay for the increased hours they need, and it simplifies administrative procedures. It raises considerably more income than assessments, but its major drawback is that the financial burden falls indiscriminately on the rich and the poor alike.

A flat rate charge of £1 per week for each client may raise five or six times the amount of an assessment system. Its effect is to reduce the cost to clients previously assessed to pay at the maximum, but it introduces charges to large numbers of clients who may previously have been assessed to pay nothing. Research in several local authorities suggests that the imposition of a standard charge causes some clients to discontinue the service: in Essex about 8 per cent of existing clients (Judge, Ferlie and Smith 1982 : 12) and in Redbridge about 10 per cent (Hyman 1980) withdrew when standard charges of £1 and £1.50 respectively were introduced.

Researchers at the University of Kent discovered that of sixty-three social services departments in England surveyed, twenty-two had introduced flat rate charges to all clients for the first time in April 1980 (Judge, Ferlie and Smith 1982 : 3). Responses to a questionnaire prepared by the West Sussex County Council showed that eleven English counties made a flat rate charge to all clients in 1980/81; three Welsh counties made a flat rate charge which was abated for clients in receipt of supplementary benefit.

A survey of home help clients undertaken by Cheshire County Council revealed that of those receiving a free service 20 per cent said they would not be willing to pay a standard charge of £1 a week. The researchers estimated that 43 per cent of those unwilling to pay would not manage satisfactorily and would 'probably find life very difficult without the home help service' (Cheshire Social Services Department 1980 : para. 4.1.3).

Despite the increased number of clients receiving accounts under a flat rate charge, accounting procedures can be simplified because each client pays the same amount. This has led to some authorities arranging for the introduction of special home help stamps which can be purchased at post offices when social security payments are made, so that clients are spared the trouble and expense of sending their remittance by post. The home help then submits the stamps with her time sheet or other documentation to her organiser. The post office makes an administrative charge to the authority concerned: nineteen local authorities had special arrangements of this kind with the post office in 1982. Once an arrangement of this kind has been instituted, it is difficult to make changes in the event of the post office charge increasing.

A standard charge can be combined with the assessment of clients on higher incomes. This raises more income but retains all the drawbacks of the assessment system, in that it requires organisers to seek information about income and outgoings.

The reader may feel that charging systems are so complex that it is difficult if not impossible to ensure that any particular system achieves the political and financial objectives it is designed to meet. It is not known with any certainty how the incidence of charges on clients in different circumstances varies with different systems. If home help services were provided by commercial undertakings, one or more specialist companies would have emerged by now to provide advice on what particular assessment and charging methods would achieve given financial objectives. Expert companies already exist to advise organisations on how to obtain maximum benefit from electricity tariffs and how to reduce telephone costs. A research project financed by the local authority associations or the Department of Health and Social Security, and aimed at establishing the impact on clients and on income of different assessment systems, would be a worthwhile investment. As the Department of Health and Social Security noted in 1973, 'The whole area of financial assessment, for whom, by whom and on what sort of scale, is one which seems to need attention'. The issue was put more prosaically in the Minority Report of the Royal Commission on the Poor Law before the first world war – and the problem has remained essentially the same since the nineteenth century.

10 · The management task

Previous chapters have indicated some of the constraints that must be taken into account in both the planning and operation of the service. We now consider in more detail the tasks of managers in social services departments, and how they ensure that the constraints of finance, manpower, staff training, and employment legislation are moderated to provide a cost-effective service to clients and ratepayers.

ELECTED MEMBERS

The management of public services differs from most other forms of management in that accountability is to a randomly selected group of individuals elected by the people, and not to persons with particular skills, or knowledge of management, or of the service being provided. The distinctive quality of the elected member is his capacity to represent the views and wishes of his electorate. He may, of course, possess work skills that relate to the functions of local government, and he may have a flair for management. Nevertheless, his special contribution to the operation of local government lies in his representative role.

The elected member's loyalty to his party and to his local electorate is likely to be greater than his loyalty to the council on which he sits or to the staff his council employs. His key task is to serve the people who have entrusted him with power; their assessment of his performance, and that of his colleagues, will determine his political future, so their aspirations are infinitely more important to him than those of local government officers. Yet the elected member must forge a working relationship with staff since it is they who supply him with information and advice and who carry out the policies he seeks to achieve. The elected member, then, is on a seesaw, first identifying with his constituency and then with the bureaucracy of government. Mutual give-and-take between officers and members should ensure that the seesaw keeps on the move and does not settle into the ground at either end.

The system by which local government officers are accountable to elected representatives creates some unique management problems. For example, there is pressure on an elected member to ensure that his constituents receive a good service from the authority. When he learns of an elector requiring a service, whether it be a home help, admission to a residential home, or some other service, he will be tempted to ask staff to divert resources so that the need can be met regardless of overall priorities. This situation can only be resolved by detailed discussion of needs, resources, and priorities between the elected representative and staff; in most instances there emerges a mutual respect that officers and members perform different roles and are consequently subjected to different pressures.

When problems arise within services, and public criticisms ensue, elected members are severely tested. As part of the council, with overall responsibility for services, they must accept responsibility for failures, yet they also identify with the public and with their electorate, who may be critical of the way in which services are operated. The temptation for elected members to disassociate themselves from problems and to scapegoat staff is very great. Sometimes, of course, staff are at fault and fail to carry out their duties properly, but there are occasions when criticisms occur after elected members have taken decisions contrary to the advice of their officers. For example, the social services committee may have devoted fewer resources to a particular service than recommended, or may have rejected proposals for an improved management structure, rendering the service badly managed.

The level of resources devoted to social services departments can be a highly political issue, but beyond that members on many social services committees act in unison with differences of view crossing political boundaries. However, in some authorities an opposition party may decide, particularly just before an election, that there are advantages in a campaign that denigrates the service. While errors of fact can and must be corrected, local government officers generally find it best to keep a low profile when their service is used as the battleground for a political dog-fight. An officer whose views appear to show allegiance to one party on such occasions will lose the respect of all. It can be an uncomfortable experience to witness destructive criticism of a service, but it seldom lasts long; it can, however, damage relationships between staff and elected members.

Members of local authorities bear a corporate responsibility for their actions. Although committee chairmen or party spokesmen may appear to carry special responsibilities, they possess no executive powers unless specifically authorised by a committee; even in such circumstances any decisions they make must be ratified by the council or by a committee of the council with delegated responsibilities.

Whilst changes in policy, particularly those requiring increased expenditure, must first be formally considered by at least one committee of elected members, it is important to recognise the informal role played by various pressure groups, by trade unions, by senior local authority managers, and by the machinery of party politics in producing a climate for change. Elected members who are committed to the development of a particular service will seek information to support their cause in discussions within their own party, as well as for public debate in committee meetings and on the hustings. They must not only be able to put forward a good case for more expenditure, they must convince their political colleagues that the service they wish to expand is in greater need of development than others and that the electorate will be prepared to meet the cost.

Thus it is important for managers at all levels in a social services department to ensure that comprehensive information is available to elected members about social needs in the locality, the way they are being met, and the shortfall in provision. Unless this information, constantly updated, is given to them, they do not have the basic tools they need to protect and develop the service.

PROFESSIONAL ASPECTS

Whilst the role of managers is broadly the same in whatever organisation they work, there are specific functions related to the nature of different organisations and the tasks they perform that make it difficult for managers to interchange between services. The management of caring tasks requires managers who are skilled and knowledgeable in those tasks so that decisions are sensitive to the needs and objectives of the organisation. For convenience we call these aspects of the management task in the home help service *professional*.

Certain principles of good management apply irrespective of the professional context. Most research into management has been carried out in commercial and industrial undertakings, and it has sometimes been difficult to appreciate the relevance of research findings to public services. However, with the growth of the public sector and the development of large-scale organisations it has become increasingly necessary for public services to learn from experience elsewhere and to foster its own research.

Sometimes clients, because of the nature of their problems or of their personalities, present unusual difficulties for the service. For example, they may reduce a steady succession of home helps to tears by their behaviour; they may complain constantly to their member of parliament or local councillor about poor or inadequate levels of service; they may cause concern because of their obvious inability to cope during the hours when the home help is not available; they may be the subject of complaints and pressure from neighbours. It is not reasonable to expect local managers to make decisions on difficult cases of this kind. There must be a framework of discussion for deciding upon them. Local managers need to feel that the decision they have made will be understood and supported by more senior staff in the event of a complaint. On some occasions it may be necessary to inform the director of social services of problems that may explode onto the political scene, and he in turn may consult a committee chairman. Whilst action of this kind is no insurance against public criticism and personal attack, it is important to ensure that there is full discussion of complex cases and that local managers feel supported by their seniors when they are criticised.

Liaison arrangements with other services, both within the social services department and beyond, are an important aspect of a home help manager's role. At senior levels there should be regular meetings with representatives of social work, medical, and nursing services to discuss policy issues, planning for the future, and co-operative working arrangements; these meetings need to be replicated at local level, so that the home help organiser can feel herself to be part of an overall caring team in her locality and can be made aware of the problems and shortcomings as they arise.

The service frequently comes under serious attack from people who have not understood the nature of the service or its limitations. The fact that home helps do not operate from an office and that they largely work alone creates management problems of a complexity that are seldom encountered in other services. The organiser cannot look round the office to see who is working that day; nor can she rely on an on-site foreman to telephone her with information about who has attended for work that morning. She is dependent for information on home helps themselves telephoning the office if they are unable to work, and she may not be able to locate a replacement before the client, his relatives, or an interested professional telephones to complain.

As more and more home helps have telephones installed in their homes and more have access to cars, it is possible to plug gaps in the service more readily than in former years, but an influenza epidemic can still play havoc with the workloading arranged by an organiser. The logistics of domiciliary services are often ill-understood by professionals who undertook their training in hospitals and in other institutions. A temporary staff shortage in hospital means that available staff are spread more thinly and that some tasks of less importance for some patients are not undertaken. Temporary staff shortage in a domiciliary service, however, means that certain clients will not receive a service at all; and although the organiser will endeavour to switch her home helps around, so that the most needy clients receive a service, such arrangements may take time to make and some clients with very great needs will be neglected.

Whilst the re-allocation of home helps between clients is necessary to ensure that those with the greatest needs receive priority, the very act of transferring staff leads to another series of complaints and criticisms from clients, their relatives, and other professionals. The home help service is a very individual and personal service. The client who lets a stranger into her home to undertake everyday tasks is likely to feel apprehensive; a good home help seeks to forge a friendly personal relationship with the client. Not only is the client upset when a new face appears on the scene, but the home help herself may feel upset that she is suddenly moved without discussion. The trauma can be minimised if full explanations are given to the client and to the home help, but the pressure of time rarely makes this possible.

Whilst it is usually helpful to ensure that the client receives a continuity of service from the same home help, the admission of a client to hospital makes it necessary to transfer the home help to another client in need. When the first client returns home after a few weeks it requires a judgement of Solomon to decide whether the original home help should be restored, or whether another should be allocated. If the original home help is allocated the second client may feel let down, but if she is not the first client may feel rejected – to the extent of making things difficult for her new home help. Like the policeman's, the home help organiser's lot is not always a happy one: she must frequently choose between two unpopular courses of action and then defend her decision.

There are advantages in retaining some home helps to deal with emergencies, especially those that arise because of staff absences. With a large workforce unforeseen absences will constantly occur which must be covered by deploying other available staff. The presence of a small number of emergency home helps, who can be assigned as necessary each morning, makes this task easier.

Another source of criticism and complaint concerns the timescale which is required for the service to respond to requests for home help. Clients, their relatives, and staff in the health service frequently complain that the home help service is not available for the first three or four days after a patient's discharge home from hospital; it is known that it is during this period that the need for care is greatest. This is a serious problem and many changes have been made in the service to make it more responsive to the needs of discharged patients. However, if it is to work effectively there must be a full understanding from other professionals of the needs of the service. A telephone call at 4 p.m. on Friday to the effect that a patient has just left a hospital and is in urgent need of a home help is a reflection of the way in which some hospitals are organised.

Although a small number of local authorities provide emergency services which can be contacted at evenings and weekends and offer a prompt response, it is not reasonable to expect the service to provide emergency cover in respect of circumstances that can be plainly foreseen. Given adequate warning of the intention to discharge a patient from hospital, an organiser can assess the need, notify a home help, and ensure that, if necessary, a service is provided from the moment the patient arrives home. Emergency services should be reserved for unforeseen problems; it is not realistic to expect more than a small number of home helps to be on call at all times, and it would be financially ruinous to make them available in such numbers that they could respond to telephone calls on the day of hospital discharge.

Much criticism and complaint can be forestalled by ensuring that allied professions and the public generally recognise the limitations of the service. Also, a readiness to respond promptly to queries and complaints from clients and their relatives will help to avoid disputes and disagreements developing into formal complaints against the authority. Inevitably, however, there are occasions when clients, or those acting on their behalf, feel that the service has not responded appropriately. It is important that procedures are established to ensure that formal complaints against the decision of an organiser are fully and impartially investigated, and that a speedy response is sent to the complainant.

Complaints come to notice in a number of ways. Sometimes the organiser at local level is telephoned by the client or a relative and told that a decision she has made is unsatisfactory or that the service being supplied is inadequate. Immediate discussion of the situation may lead to an early resolution to the satisfaction of all parties, but it is important that administrative machinery exists to review the matter at a more senior level if agreement cannot be reached. This machinery should enable a complaint to be referred to elected members in the event of continual dissatisfaction.

Unfortunately, few complaints proceed through the paths designed for them. Often clients complain to their councillors and members of parliament, the local press, the chief executive, the director of social services, or another member of staff, without making it clear to their local organiser that they are dissatisfied with the service. A good deal of correspondence to, from, and within social services departments is taken up with redirecting queries, appeals, and complaints that bypass staff with appropriate delegated authority. This should not mislead the reader into believing that there are significant numbers of complaints about the operation of social services departments. In the course of a year a large department may be responsible for over half a million home help visits. If one contact in 20,000 proves unsatisfactory to the extent that a member of the public makes a formal complaint, this represents about twenty-five complaints per year – which would be regarded as very high.

That few complaints are received about the operation of the personal social services, despite rising public expectations, results from a com-bination of two factors: high standards among staff who deal directly with the public, and a natural fear on the part of people who rely on public services that if they complain the service will be withdrawn altogether. The absence of clear and enforceable rights places clients at the mercy of professional staff, who must always be sensitive to this fact.

In most instances complaints that reach a social services department via a councillor or member of parliament can be resolved at local level; such complaints often relate to a decision to refuse or to discontinue a service, but can also include complaints about individual home helps who are said to be late for work, leave early, are rude, dishonest, or do poor work. Where dissatisfaction persists, despite engaging in discussion at local level, it is important that full consideration is given to the matter at a more senior level in the department.

The introduction of formal complaints procedures within local authorities was given a stimulus by the creation of the Commission for Local Administration in England (colloquially named the local govern-ment ombudsman) under the Local Government Act of 1974. Both the commission and a government report on conduct in local government (Redcliffe-Maud Committee 1974) urged local authorities to formulate and publicise complaints procedures. The Personal Social Services Council published a paper on this subject in 1976 with model procedures for social services departments, and two years later the Commission for Local Administration, in association with a representative body of local authorities, agreed a code of practice for local authorities to follow. As a consequence there can be few local authorities that have not devised their own formal complaints procedures.

The local government ombudsman is, in a sense, a long stop; she is not, however, a substitute for proper scrutiny of decision-taking within social services departments. The powers of the ombudsman are limited. She cannot enquire into the merits of a professional decision but only into the manner in which that decision was taken. She will take into account such factors as unfairness, bias, incompetence, or excessive delay, but will not attempt to determine whether the decision reached by an authority was right or wrong. For example, the ombudsman may conclude that there was maladministration because the social services department took too long to reach a decision, because it did not keep the client informed of what was happening, or that it reached a decision without first carrying out a full and proper assessment. Despite the narrowness of her role and the fact that few social services complaints are received and investigated, the local government ombudsman has ensured that staff in social services departments and elected representatives are much more aware of the need to formalise complaints procedures and to deal meticulously and seriously with all complaints received. Although a finding of guilt by the ombudsman does not represent total humiliation, no one – staff or elected member – wants his service publicly discredited by an adverse report.

The provision of in-service training for organisers and home helps is a key task for all managers in the service. Senior staff also have a responsibility to ensure that liaison is maintained with local training institutions so that relevant short courses are made available. It is important, too, that each home help service has an established policy about seconding suitable staff on training courses, leading to a qualification in home help organisation.

A disturbing feature of professionalism in the caring services is the way in which each separate profession develops a blinkered and stereotyped view of the rest. The houseman or registrar who fails to secure a home help for a patient he discharges from hospital at a moment's notice is unlikely to appreciate the reasons and may harbour a dislike of the service for many years thereafter, believing it to be inefficient and incapable of responding to the needs of his patients. It is, therefore, important that managers in the home help service are made available to lecture to other professional groups both during their professional training and on refresher courses. It is also mutually beneficial if student doctors, nurses, administrators, occupational therapists, social workers, and others spend part of their training in a social services department, working alongside home help organisers and learning the nature of their jobs at first hand.

FINANCIAL AND ADMINISTRATIVE ISSUES

The administrative functions of home help organisers and other managers in social services departments should ensure that services operate within the policies decided upon, and that resources in terms of money and staff skills are used efficiently and to the best effect. Professional and administrative functions are not separate entities. It is common for professional staff employed in large organisations to criticise the administration for placing restrictions on them, but all professional staff who have control over resources carry out administrative functions and there are always limitations to professional practice. Administration is as much enabling as restricting; it concerns the orderly use of a range of resources to meet agreed objectives.

Managers have a key part to play in the preparation of the annual budget. Their first aim must be to ensure that the budgetary provision enables current policies to be pursued. Each year they should review expenditure under a variety of headings such as salaries, wages, equipment, clothing, and travelling costs, so that the social services committee can be informed of the level of service that can be provided in the year ahead. The committee then has an opportunity to seek additional funds from the authority if it feels it can argue a strong enough case against the competing demands of other committees. Alternatively, the social services committee may decide to reallocate sums between budget heads under its own control, and so permit the growth of the home help service by transferring money from some other service.

A given level of expenditure will only buy a certain amount of service. For the social services committee to make intelligent decisions when the annual budget is under consideration, it must have a clear idea of the nature and extent of the present service as well as the extent of unmet need.

Once the annual budget is established, managers must monitor expenditure throughout the year. It is not intrinsically wrong for a budget to be over- or underspent in the course of the year. What *is* important is that the trend is identified at an early stage, the reasons for it are understood, and either expenditure patterns are corrected to correspond with the original budget or, if this will have an important impact on the provision of services, the social services committee is invited to review the position. Even during periods when local authorities are expanding their services, it is difficult for a social services committee to secure additional finance from a finance committee during the course of the year. Over-expenditure must therefore normally be corrected, either by reducing costs or by transferring money from another budget head.

In a service as extensive as the home help service, where management decisions are made by a great number of people in various offices, there must be a delegation of administrative decisions in a way that gives field managers clear responsibilities within the framework of a unified policy for the department as a whole. For example, there may be a sum in the budget to cover the travelling expenses of home helps. It will be the task of senior managers in the department to allocate this sum between all the home help organisers, bearing in mind that the expenditure incurred under this heading will vary between different areas. Each local organiser will endeavour to keep within her allocation, but senior managers will examine statistical returns in the course of the year to be satisfied that the budget is being properly expended. A combination of circumstances in a particular area may cause claims for travelling costs to rise sharply; this may be due to an increase in clients or home helps living in remote parts. If the increased expenditure appears reasonable to the senior manager, she will try to transfer sums from other areas that may not be fully spending their budget allocation; however, if expenditure is generally high on this item she may need to place artificial restrictions on travelling expenses, or seek to transfer sums from other budget heads that she believes will be underspent or she regards as covering less important expenditure. Such a step would normally be discussed with a manager responsible for a wider span of control because it might be felt appropriate to transfer money from a budget head outside the home help service.

Wages form the biggest part of the home help budget. The steady turnover of home helps and the variety of hours they work make it important to create a simple method of control to ensure that local organisers have the maximum freedom to recruit and to plan work within the overall sum allocated to them. This can be done fairly simply by converting the sum in the budget to an equivalent number of hours and allocating these hours between all the organisers operating at local level. An organiser allocated 26,000 hours of home-help time during the course of a year would know that this enabled her to employ an average of 500 hours each week. Inevitably the number of hours employed fluctuates; it may be difficult to fill vacancies as they arise, or it may be considered appropriate to reduce services slightly in the summer months in order to provide more intensity in the winter. Account must be taken of premium payments for overtime working, so that if a group of home helps receives more than the hourly rate this is taken into account by the organiser in calculating the remaining hours available to her.

Such a system of budget allocation gives maximum flexibility to the local manager and helps to ensure that large sums of money are not left unspent at the end of a financial year. However, there are limitations. The organiser who finds that she has unspent money in her budget towards the end of the financial year will be cautious about engaging more staff, for this will mean that she starts the new year with a commitment for staff wages that cannot be sustained; in order to redress this commitment she would feel obliged not to replace staff when they left, yet the pattern of resignations across her area might not be consistent with the needs of clients requiring a service. Only by careful control throughout the year and intelligent anticipation can the organiser ensure that her service is responsive to local needs and that she makes the best use of the money available.

Local authorities adopt a variety of policies and practices with regard to income and expenditure in the home help service. When financial assessments of clients are undertaken they are usually processed by organisers, but the preparation of accounts and the pursuit of defaulters are sometimes placed in the hands of staff in the treasurer's department. Where charges are based on an assessment of the client's ability to pay, a system of time sheets for home helps is essential to ensure that the client is charged only for the hours worked. The checking of time sheets is an expensive operation in itself, and in some authorities where standard charges are levied or the service is free they have been abandoned altogether. Nevertheless, administrative systems are required to record the number of hours worked by each home help, including any overtime that has been authorised. This information, together with facts about annual leave arrangements and sickness, must be forwarded to the staff responsible for calculating and paying wages. Most home helps are paid weekly, although in the County of Avon considerable financial savings were made when monthly payments were introduced. Staff engaged in special schemes such as family aides or home aides are often employed on officer grades and are paid monthly.

There is no consistent way in which travelling time and travelling expenses are treated. Audrey Hunt found in 1967 that nearly 90 per cent of local authorities paid home helps for the time spent travelling between clients (Hunt 1970 : 333). It is arguable whether time taken to travel to the first case of the day and back home from the last case should qualify for payment, since it is not normal for employers to pay staff for their travelling time to and from work. However, where arrangements are made for a home help to travel at a distance from her home, special consideration may be required. Whilst there can be no doubt that home helps should be paid appropriate travelling expenses between cases, practices differ about meeting expenses to the first case and home from the last.

To save time and to provide a more responsive service some local authorities are prepared to meet car expenses for home helps. Proportionately few home helps have access to a car, but the presence of two or three highly mobile home helps on a team greatly eases the task of an organiser, particularly when emergencies arise. It is important, however, that home helps do not begin to feel that those with cars are given special privileges. Some authorities provide mopeds for home helps to reduce travelling time and to aid mobility. Whilst such arrangements can add to the effectiveness of the service they entail additional responsibilities for organisers.

Audrey Hunt found that most local authorities provided special clothing for home helps, although the items supplied varied, including overalls, coats, caps, and aprons; a small number supplied rubber gloves (Hunt 1970 : 51). The issuing of clothing, face masks (for households with infectious diseases), and other items of protective clothing presents problems of control to organisers. Clearly such items must be issued whenever needed with the minimum amount of formality, yet checks must be made to ensure that there is no abuse.

Views differ about whether home helps should be supplied with distinctive clothing in the form of a recognisable uniform. A well-designed overall or dress can add status and even glamour to the service. The airlines have discovered how to make a mundane task such as serving food and drink to passengers into a highly sought-after career: they have achieved this by providing attractive uniforms and adopting the glamorous title *air hostess*. Home helps perform much more interesting, varied, and vital work than air hostesses; although this is not reflected in their pay, it is possible to provide them with a uniform they can wear with pride. This helps to render them more recognisable to community nurses, general practitioners, and other persons providing domiciliary care.

Some households in which home helps work are deficient in cleaning materials and equipment. Clients are expected to make satisfactory provision, but a home help must be able to turn to her employer for assistance if the client is unable or unwilling to provide the bare essentials. Whatever arrangements are made by the organiser to provide cleaning materials, there is an element of bureaucracy in the control arrangements that will be inconvenient and irksome to home helps. For small items, reimbursement from petty cash is probably the most satisfactory arrangement, although if the small sums become large some restrictions may be necessary; many home helps supply their own materials and fail to claim reimbursement from the authority.

Some authorities have a supply of larger items such as vacuum cleaners, but unless transport is provided or the home help herself travels by car the arrangements necessary to use them are cumbersome and time-consuming; these problems are not easy to overcome without considerable expenditure. The supply of small shopping trolleys can be helpful if they enable home helps to undertake shopping for two or three clients at the same time.

Statistics are a basic tool for managers. By collecting the right statistics and comparing them over periods of time and between different geographical areas, the skilful manager can detect changing patterns and plan accordingly. Statistics of course do not tell the whole story, for each figure represents a unique human problem, but figures can form the basis for considering change. The individual home help may become aware that the clients to whom she is allotted are more frail and dependent than in former years, but she will not know whether this is a developing feature of the service or whether it is due to chance. The first-line organiser, on the other hand, will be able to build up a picture of the service in her locality over a period of time and assess what changes are taking place; she may then be able to compare her findings with the experience of other areas both inside and outside her own local authority.

At more senior levels in a social services department, statistics of the home help service may be studied alongside those of other services, such as home nursing, or admissions to geriatric care or elderly persons' homes. This may reveal a changing pattern of care which, in turn, should be reflected in the way in which the home help service is managed.

Reliable information about services is very difficult to assemble unless it is collated routinely as part of basic record-keeping at local level. Most staff in social services departments find the collection of statistical information a painful chore. It is not useful information until it is collated, presented, analysed, and compared with information gathered elsewhere or at other times; only after these procedures does the raw information fed into the system by large numbers of organisers and clerks become a valuable commodity, capable of revealing changes occurring among the population in need and the way in which the service is being provided. Without this information it is not possible to plan effectively for the future or to convince local authority committees (which have immense pressure on them to release more resources for every conceivable aspect of their work) that the service should be expanded.

The collection and interpretation of statistical material about the personal social services presents immense problems. The reasons why clients need a service can be recorded, in many instances, under two or more different headings. It was noted in Chapter 2 that the number of families receiving a home help due to the presence of a mentally handicapped adult was understated in Department of Health and Social Security statistics, because where the parents were aged over 65 help was classified as for the elderly. There are various ways of classifying the purpose of the help offered to families with multiple problems. The presence of mental illness, alcoholism, physical illness, or under-developed children may all be considered of significance, and it may be a matter of chance how the family is shown in statistical returns. Where the choice is difficult there is a tendency to classify according to the nature of the organisation that first requested the help. This all points to the need for careful interpretation of statistical returns. The problem is not confined to the United Kingdom. At an international seminar a German observer quoted an organiser who said she registered families 'under the organisation footing the bill' (Jonas 1975 : 8).

Statistical information gathered within the service can sometimes be used with specific studies to demonstrate that new approaches to old and familiar problems might be cost effective. Most social services depart-ments have small groups of staff who undertake research work. Some have co-operated with home help organisers and their staff to produce valuable information about the operation of the service, revealing the attitudes of clients to different charging policies, the extent to which emergency services are required, or the growth in services needed to avoid unnecessary admissions to elderly persons' homes.

Managers in the service must ensure that all the paraphernalia of modern office systems are available and properly used. Staff require adequate furniture and equipment and need to have facilities to operate administrative systems. Special attention must be paid to telephones since so much communication between the organiser, her clients, and home helps takes place on the telephone. It is preferable for each organiser to have a direct telephone line that does not pass through the departmental telephone exchange, so that she can be contacted with relative ease from a public telephone box. There must be adequate organisers and clerks to perform the duties required; office staff must be located appropriately to be near the clients they serve and have ease of access to other related services. It is also necessary to ensure that proper arrangements are made for answering simple enquiries and taking messages in the absence of the organiser.

Good publicity about the service is an aid to recruitment and assists the public generally to understand the purpose and nature of the service, thus helping to avoid unreal expectations. Leaflets written in straight-forward English and made available in hospitals, general practitioners' waiting-rooms, libraries, and offices of voluntary and statutory services, have the dual role of informing the general public and the voluntary and statutory staff who provide advice to clients in need. Many authorities have devised publicity material of this kind which contains information about where to apply for further details. In areas where a high proportion of the population originates from overseas, there is value in providing publicity material in ethnic minority languages.

Research studies carried out in the United Kingdom raise doubts about the capacity of organisers to manage resources appropriately. Not only have questions been raised about whether clients with the greatest needs receive effective help, there is evidence that home helps do not always carry out the duties assessed as necessary by organisers, and that a significant waste of home help hours can arise due to unnecessary travelling. Insufficient clerical support for organisers, their large span of control, the dearth of training for home helps, the fragmented nature of the service, the relative isolation of organisers from other professionals, the need for regular contact with staff from a range of services, the inadequacy of training for organisers, and the sheer unremitting burden of trying to provide a service that is sensitive to the needs of clients and responds quickly to requests for help, have all reduced the capacity of organisers to provide an ideal service.

The performance of organisers might be improved by identifying more duties that could be performed by clerks and other personnel. Professionals are not renowned for their enthusiasm to delegate functions to ancillary staff and organisers commonly delegate only routine tasks to their clerks, failing to appreciate the degree of assistance that they can provide. A study in Cumbria (Gwynne 1980) revealed that clerks were able to prevent waste and improve efficiency by the careful planning of home help allocations so that travelling time was kept to a minimum. However, there was considerable resistance by organisers to changing their ways of working. In few authorities are there sufficient clerks to enable organisers to delegate more responsibilities, but it is important that the training of organisers covers the effective deployment of clerks and other ancillary staff.

Some aspects of financial assessment and the collection of charges from clients, including bad debts and calculations about wages and expenses, are matters that can be carried out by staff with appropriate expertise outside the home help service. A good personnel section or department can provide advice and assistance to organisers by supplying specialist information and processing routine matters like advertisements for staff and the preparation of letters of appointment.

The processing of time sheets represents a massive administrative chore in many authorities. They are only strictly relevant where clients pay an hourly charge. No other public servants suffer the indignity of asking the public they visit to certify that they have received a service; it is a practice that should be discontinued.

MANAGEMENT OF PERSONNEL

Management is concerned with the effective use of resources. The home help service is labour intensive: over 90 per cent of costs are attributable to salaries and wages. Thus good personnel management is of fundamental importance in ensuring an efficient and responsive service. Failures in professional direction and in administrative systems will lead to a misuse of resources, but the best managed service will crumble unless there is a unity of purpose between staff at all levels so that those who are employed in the service feel they are important and their individuality is recognised.

A unity of purpose can only be achieved by clarifying objectives, by specifying well-defined expectations of each member of staff, and by firm direction and control. Yet this is only one side of the equation, for, unless they share the overall objectives of the organisation and understand the need for direction and control, human beings tend to resent instructions. Indeed, they need to feel that they can make a contribution towards the planning of services and influence key decisions about operational policies.

In any organisation employing personnel, staff selection is an important aspect of the management task. Poor selection, in which staff are appointed who are unable to meet the demands made upon them, leads to inefficiency and a loss of morale. Staff should be selected not merely on an assessment of their ability to meet the requirements of the job, but also with an eye to their capacity to benefit from training and to develop skills in a way that will enhance the service. High staff turnover can be very expensive. Not only is it time-consuming for organisers to be continually interviewing for new staff, but inevitably new recruits need time to settle into the work. They need instruction and training, which is expensive to provide. A stable workforce is not only more efficient than one that is constantly changing, it reduces the pressure on managers and releases their time to undertake more vital work on behalf of the service.

The best recruits are likely to be those who are recommended to apply by existing staff, or who respond following publicity about the service and its work. However, employment opportunities, particularly for part-time staff, vary throughout the country, and, depending upon local circumstances, job centres or press advertisements may be required. Organisers will need to follow whatever staff recruitment policies are laid down within the local authority in which they work. There may be centralised systems and forms for inserting advertisements, for receiving applications, for obtaining references, and for issuing letters of appointment. However, the key to good selection procedures is the interview, in which the organiser tries to learn about the applicant, her aspirations, her attitudes to people in need, and her practical ability.

Some applicants for the post of home help have little previous employment experience, and many seek a job after a considerable interval during which they have been looking after their families. Discussions may, therefore, concentrate on current family responsibilities rather than on previous work experience. The interviewer will seek to learn whether the applicant can organise herself to run a home smoothly, and whether she appears capable of adapting herself to the needs of different households. If she can be encouraged to talk about her family and her neighbours she will express her personality and reveal whether she is friendly, kindhearted, tactful, and tolerant. The organiser must assess whether the applicant is likely to be honest in her dealings with dependent people and whether she can be relied upon not to discuss private and confidential information about clients with other people.

By the end of the interview the organiser should have a clear idea of the applicant's aptitude for the work, the hours she might be able to offer, any limitations that may arise due to family commitments or difficulties in travelling, the kind of clients for which she might be best suited, and any particular issues that should be explored with the applicant during training. At this interview, and again when the applicant starts work and during induction training, as much information as possible should be imparted so that she has as full an understanding as possible about the service and what is required of her.

Ease of communication between staff can avoid or at least reduce many problems, but by the nature of the job personal contact between organisers and their home helps is difficult to sustain. Audrey Hunt (1970 : 69) found that about a quarter of home helps saw their organiser less often than once in two months; contact in country areas was less frequent than in large towns. A printed statement for each home help outlining the purpose of the service, the way in which it is organised, what tasks she will be expected to carry out, and who to contact in the event of difficulty, can be extremely valuable.

There are few opportunities for home helps to meet together as a group with their organiser. The meetings that are arranged usually take place during the home help's own time, and attendance is therefore voluntary. The staff who attend are likely to be those who are most interested in the service and who wish to discuss general matters of policy and practice; those who might be most in need of instruction and support may choose not to come. Social gatherings, particularly at Christmas, are a useful means of helping staff to identify with the organisation that employs them and can have a direct impact on morale. Also, a staff newsletter providing information about the service, changes in personnel, and including contributions from home helps themselves, can assist in breaking down barriers.

Organisers must not neglect the welfare of their workforce. The absence of regular formal contact between organisers and home helps means that personal worries, misunderstandings, and frustration may not readily come to notice. A sympathetic and understanding relationship will encourage staff to report any difficulties they are experiencing at an early stage and enable the organiser to help in any way she can. It must be emphasised that services in the United Kingdom have persistently failed to provide adequate supervision and consultation to the workforce and that, as a consequence, home helps carry considerable burdens of stress, anxiety, and even depression. They spend their working lives among people who suffer extreme privation, whose daily experiences are made wretched by physical pain, depression, and poverty, and who sometimes need to express their bitterness and despair to anyone who will listen. It is no easy task to respond positively in such circumstances, and it is clear that many home helps feel overwhelmed, unsupported, isolated, and despairing.

A home help may be desolated when a client for whom she has cared for months or years dies or suffers a serious accident; she may be overcome by a deep sense of loss and grief and express feelings of guilt, especially if death occurs when she is not in attendance. Her need to mourn may be as great as, or even greater than, that of members of the family. The figure standing on the edge of the group at the graveside during the burial service is likely to be the home help paying her last respects in her own time; she mourns alone.

The personal burdens carried by home helps in respect of their clients greatly exceed those of professional staff since they work in isolation, have few opportunities to share their concerns, are generally untrained and unprepared to deal with the impact of distress, and sustain personal contact over long periods with their clients. Phyllida Parsloe described the value for social workers of working as part of a team of colleagues: 'team members provide very considerable support for each other, and it is at least open to question whether individuals could bear the strain of their work if they were isolated from, and unsupported by, colleagues . . . the communication and support (from the team) may be a crucial factor in reducing the stress on social workers and enabling them to manage their caseloads' (1981 : 27–8). The need for personal support among home helps can be no less. Describing the intense pressures of the service, Meg Bond concluded:

'It is my contention that organisers and their home helps take on these huge burdens and fail to acknowledge openly that they are too great because they accept the ideology of housewifery which places a premium upon making do and mending, upon coping and budgeting, and upon managing within the resources available. A woman would not be a good housewife or mother, or home help or organiser, if she said she could not take responsibility for the areas which have traditionally been seen as her responsibility – housework and the care of society's dependants. To admit that she cannot meet all these demands with the resources available to her would strike at the essence of her good womanhood – at the very qualities for which the staff of the service are selected. As a result the fact is obscured that the overall level of care (as opposed to domestic service) received by the clients, is far from satisfactory. Moreover, to the extent that it is received, it is often at the cost of exploiting the home helps and creating difficulties for the staff and clients alike.' (1982 : 23)

We would like to see a greater awareness among employers and managers at all levels of the extent to which the service expects home helps to absorb the massive personal burdens of providing care.

Research suggests that job satisfaction is more likely to occur when people feel they can influence the planning and arrangement of their own work, and when duties are variable and can correspond to the various needs and aptitudes of the individuals concerned. It is helpful if employees feel a sense of common purpose, both with colleagues and supervisors, and that their work is appreciated. Such sentiments are difficult to achieve with a scattered workforce.

Various approaches have been developed in industry to involve the workforce in considerations about policy and practice. Quality Circles in Japan consist of small groups of work people who meet regularly to consider how performance can be improved and costs reduced. The mere fact of consulting practitioners and operators at local level improves communication and encourages a creative and positive approach towards the organisation, its function, and its problems. A number of major companies in the United Kingdom and the United States have built on the Japanese experience, and some local authorities have found similar methods valuable in stimulating staff to examine areas of concern.

The workforce at local level possesses considerable knowledge about practical problems, and it is important to provide opportunities for staff who wish to contribute to air their views about the service. A relaxed discussion among home helps can reveal how the provision of special clothing or equipment might improve efficiency; how a more imaginative use of local laundry facilities or community rooms might enhance the service; or how volunteers or neighbourhood groups can best assist. Home helps are the eyes and ears of the organisers. The service cannot reach its full potential unless there is respect, trust, and understanding between all those working in the service.

Apart from regular communication and discussions with staff, it is necessary to devise formal machinery for consultation and negotiation with trade unions about issues relating to working conditions, terms of service, and wages. Negotiations with trade unions normally take place on an authority-wide basis between trade union representatives and elected members. Managers from the home help service may or may not be present at such meetings, but they will wish to ensure that relevant information together with their views are made available at them. Consultation, as distinct from negotiation, usually takes place between managers and trade union representatives.

It is good practice to consult trade unions before reports concerning staffing and working conditions are considered by committees. This is desirable in order to ensure that staff views are taken into account in formulating proposals, and also to convey those views to local authority members before decisions are reached. Many local authority committees are conducted with the press and public in attendance, which means that committee decisions may be discussed in the press before there is an opportunity for the local authority formally to notify its employees of changes that have been agreed. This makes it doubly important to develop effective communication with staff and unions so that full information is provided through management channels. Consultation must be carried out with great sensitivity, because committee members will be disconcerted if they are lobbied by staff or become aware of public debates on important issues before they have received reports from the chief officer on what is proposed.

There is great value in ensuring that representatives of the workforce meet with home help managers on a regular basis to review services and to explore any difficulties that might be raised. This not only encourages the development of a mutual understanding betwen managers and home helps but can mean that problems are rectified at an early stage before they threaten to disrupt the service. People instinctively resist change, yet in a changing world services cannot stand still. Managers tend to formulate new proposals and put them into action before explaining them to the workforce and giving whatever reassurances may be necessary. The introduction of new specialist schemes, the creation of emergency services, the use of volunteers, new arrangements for co-operation with laundry services, more efficient ways of paying wages, and a host of other initiatives, may all be highly desirable, but they will have an impact on the existing workforce and it should not be assumed that everyone in the service will have the same perspective as a manager. Once issues have been fully explored and safeguards agreed, staff can be powerful allies in bringing about change and development in the service.

Home help organisers must be quick to deal not only with complaints from clients, but also with grievances expressed by home helps themselves. They may feel that their wages have been wrongly calculated, that their full expenses have not been met, that compared with colleagues they are more likely to be allocated to dirty households or to households containing clients with unsavoury habits. Such queries and complaints must be investigated promptly, thoroughly, and impartially. Local authorities have established official procedures whereby a grievance from a member of staff, if unresolved at local level, is considered by a senior manager and, if necessary, by a sub-committee of elected members. Such formal procedures are rarely used and are no substitute for good mutual understanding between the local organiser and the home helps she controls.

Inevitably some home helps prove unsatisfactory. Good practice, as well as employment legislation, demands that staff whose performance gives rise to concern are given opportunities to explain their actions and to defend themselves against accusations. If specific problems are identified it may be necessary to provide special instruction or supervision in order to overcome them. In consultation with trade unions all local authorities have adopted codes of practice that must be strictly followed where a serious breach of discipline occurs. These codes usually allow for official warnings and final warnings to be given to erring staff, and for dismissal in the event of continuing misconduct or serious breakdowns of discipline.

Staff who are believed to have committed a serious act of indiscipline may be suspended from duty pending full enquiries being undertaken. Suspension is not, in itself, an act of discipline, although inevitably it is often seen by staff as an indication that the authority has already reached firm conclusions about guilt and where it lies. Serious allegations made to the police by clients or their relatives may lead to a home help being interviewed without the knowledge of the organiser, who may then find it necessary to suspend the home help from work while further enquiries are made.

Disciplinary procedures are necessarily cumbersome and time-consuming and are generally avoided by managers if at all possible. It is, however, important to adhere to certain basic standards. If it is known that bad workmanship, poor time-keeping, false financial claims, and other forms of dishonesty, lead to no more than a few harsh words, morale within the service will suffer. Managers sometimes avoid formal disciplinary procedures because they take place in an emotionally charged atmosphere. Disciplinary hearings themselves are quite formal and follow an adversarial approach, with the member of staff being permitted to be represented by a trade union official or solicitor.

Disciplinary interviews must be conducted in a scrupulously fair way, not merely to ensure that the member of staff has a proper hearing, but also because it is important that staff generally respect the impartiality of procedures that can be applied to them. A member of staff who feels he has been treated unjustly can appeal to a committee of elected members who, after reviewing all the issues and hearing both sides, may decide to quash the findings of the disciplinary hearing. It is, therefore, important that organisers not only have their facts right but that they follow the established procedures in every detail. Nothing is more damaging to the service, or indeed to an individual organiser, than to know that, because of a failure by management fully to observe a disciplinary code of practice, dishonest home helps continue in employment.

The number of managerial posts in the home help service is generally insufficient to provide a cost-effective service. A forward-looking authority will wish to ensure that the service is directed principally towards the most vulnerable and towards rehabilitative functions. This requires a skilled assessment of need and periodic reviews to re-assess priority; the rapid turnover of clients such a policy entails places a high workload on organisers and their clerks. The need to ensure that staff appreciate the necessity of encouraging self-help in clients increases the volume of work for managers and demands greater commitment and skill. Research into caseload management would undoubtedly reveal that, in contrast to industrial and commercial organisations and, indeed, most other areas of public employment, the home help service, with its uniquely complex management problems, pays its managers badly and has fewer of them to develop and maintain the service at peak efficiency. The fact that this is principally a women's service is undoubtedly the main reason for such a state of affairs.

11 · Achieving
integrated care

The drive to reform the organisation of the United Kingdom social welfare services in the late 1960s and early 1970s was largely fuelled by the belief that social work was an unrealised resource and that, given an opportunity to unify and manage its own development, it would meet social needs more effectively. Social work was seen as the central pivot of the new departments, identifying and assessing needs and deploying a range of related services to meet them. The white paper that heralded reform in Scotland, *Social Work and the Community*, listed six reasons why a reorganisation of services was necessary; five related specifically to social work (Scottish Education Department 1966 : 3).

Field social workers have played a major role in building social welfare services despite representing only about 10 per cent of the total workforce in social services and social work departments. Nevertheless, a great many activities other than social work take place within social welfare services and it is a matter for debate whether all social welfare should be organised, managed, and supervised by social work staff. Because of a preoccupation with the role and function of social workers, their training, and their supervision, less attention has been given to organisational and training issues relating to other major groups of staff.

The Barclay working party reported in 1982 on the role and tasks of social workers. The report suggested that one of the principal tasks of social workers was 'social care planning' which it described as 'creating, with a client, a system or network of care, tailored to his particular situation' (Barclay Report 1982 : 39). The working party felt this task had in the past received too little recognition and that it tended to be dismissed as work that was of less importance than that carried out directly with clients. This perhaps reveals the dilemma about the organisation of domiciliary services. Even the word 'professional' carries the image of one who achieves his goals by face-to-face contact with clients, offering counselling and specialist advice. Whilst this is an essential role, the overwhelming need in domiciliary services is for professionals who are prepared to negotiate with a range of resource providers, including informal carers, voluntary organisations, and statutory services, to create integrated packages of care to suit the needs of individual clients and to maintain a shared responsibility for the care provided. Not only is there a tendency, as the Barclay Report suggests, for this kind of work to be regarded as requiring less skill, but those who engage in it as a principal activity, such as home help organisers, are afforded lower status as a consequence.

A critic of the Barclay working party and its terms of reference observed that the report reflected the assumption of the centrality of social work in social services departments and 'its dominance as the ruling professional ideology' (Beresford 1982 : 50). Although the report suggested that social workers had an important role to play in ensuring that client needs were met by a range of services, it made only fleeting reference to the home help service and did so in the context of home helps being ancillary to social workers; organisers were not mentioned and there was no explanation about how the two services might be managed and co-ordinated.

One forthright but untypical response to the Barclay Report came from a director of social services who said, 'The idea of the profession of an élite of social workers with a host of ancillaries on a medical model is a spurious one' (Bessell 1982 : 18). We agree that it is spurious, but the practice of medicine has moved forward from the rigid hierarchical systems of organisation of an earlier age into multi-disciplinary teams, and we believe social services departments should do the same.

The evidence of the Association of Directors of Social Services to the Barclay working party indicated that social workers often worked 'in concert' with home helps and felt that, ideally, 'all requests to a social services department should be seen by a social worker' (1982 : 19, 58), but did not follow this through with a discussion about the role of organisers or their relationship with social workers. Goldberg and Connelly have suggested that social workers should ensure that 'different support services function adequately and in an integrated fashion' (1982 : 89), and have explained that research studies showed that 'most elderly clients who come to the attention of social workers in area offices will be assessed, receive some advice and information and be put in touch with appropriate forms of practical help' (p.94). Like the Barclay working party, Goldberg and Connelly do not specify how an assessment by social workers compares with an assessment carried out by a home help organiser, and do not discuss the relationship between these two groups of staff.

Research findings do not support the widespread assumption that field social workers play a central controlling and supervising role in the provision of domiciliary care for the elderly. A number of studies have shown that qualified social workers prefer working with children and families rather than with the elderly, and that untrained social workers and welfare assistants are more likely to provide help for the elderly than their qualified colleagues.

Many people requiring practical support are seen by social workers or social work assistants and then, following an assessment of need, are referred to a home help organiser who undertakes a further assessment and, depending on work priorities, decides whether or not service can be offered. A considerable number of elderly clients – probably the majority – are referred to organisers direct without being assessed by social workers. This may arise because a doctor, nurse, or other person specifies that a home help is required, or because an outline of the circumstances by telephone or in a letter to the department signifies that the allocation of a home help is likely to represent the appropriate response. In many authorities, occupational therapists also receive and investigate both direct and indirect requests for assistance, mainly in relation to the elderly and handicapped. Thus social services departments commonly employ three different categories of professional staff who each assess the needs of clients for domiciliary care.

In the absence of a co-ordinated approach to the assessment of need, there is a danger that each professional will define and assess needs according to his own skills and according to the services he controls. There is a clear need for co-ordinated work, and this has led some observers to urge that social workers should colonise staff from other professional groups.

Social work and home help services have traditionally been regarded as separate areas of domiciliary care, providing distinctive but complementary care. Whilst they commonly cover coterminous geographical areas and sometimes share administrative systems, there is seldom close dialogue between social workers and organisers except where special schemes have brought them together to formulate jointly agreed policies, or where senior managers have taken particular care to encourage close working arrangements. Integrated care has been a chimera. Even when new and exciting collaborative schemes have been developed, staff in adjacent offices may be unaware of them and therefore untouched by the potential for joint initiatives. Even the reading matter of social workers and organisers is likely to follow separate and predictable paths. They largely attend separate conferences; their professional associations barely communicate, while tensions and inter-professional rivalry are easily discernible in a mixed gathering of social workers and organisers.

Unfortunately, differences in the origin of the two services in organisation, in structure, in training, and in work content have all conspired to encourage a belief among practitioners that a gulf between the perceptions of social workers and organisers is inevitable. Difficulties in identifying ways of bringing greater unity to the two services without the trauma that would accompany any attempt to make one service subservient to the other mean that the two services generally run in parallel with a minimum of communication between them.

The uncertain relationship between home help organisers and social workers is reminiscent of the subdued hostility between some social workers and medical officers in the 1950s and 1960s. At that time, it was common for social workers to complain that their training and ability were not recognised or appreciated by medical staff. Ashdown and Brown described the failure of some psychiatrists 'to understand what psychiatric social workers have been trained to undertake' (1953 : 143). Marjorie Ward referred to 'the reluctance of many medical officers of health to recognise the need for trained and expert personnel' in social work (1960 : 124).

Writing in 1964 about the need to combine all local authority social welfare services under one chief officer, a medical officer of health complained that social work staff were unfitted to run social welfare services because 'their outlook on social problems will be restricted only to their experience in their particular field' (Thompson 1964 : 87). He felt that medical officers of health alone possessed the necessary training and experience. The Seebohm Committee declared that mutual mis-understanding between medical officers of health and social workers 'has gone so far as to be a significant factor in our overall thinking on the future shape of the social services'; the report went on 'but the situation is at its worst in general practice' (Seebohm Committee 1968 : 213). Thus inter-professional rivalry was an important consideration in establishing the administrative separation of medical and social work services.

It is ironic that the kind of criticism levelled by social workers about doctors in the past is now applied by organisers to social workers, and that the response by social workers to the emerging profession of home help organiser mirrors that adopted by doctors towards social work when it was struggling for a professional identity. Hedley and Norman (1982 : 26) found that half the organisers they interviewed were dissatisfied with their relationship with social workers. Organisers said they found social workers difficult to work with, and that they made decisions without consulting organisers or home helps who sometimes possessed considerable knowledge about the client and his circumstances. There are significant differences in perception between organisers and social workers about the nature and potential of the service. Perhaps that is why a Northern Ireland study found that home helps saw their training needs in terms of personal and social care, whereas social work staff felt that home help training should concentrate on household tasks (Central Personal Social Services Advisory Committee 1981 : 36).

Pressure to redefine the relationship between social workers and organisers arises from two connected issues. First, attempts to provide an intensive service for clients with high needs have made it increasingly obvious that the skills of both groups of staff are required in a collaborative approach if domiciliary care is to be a real alternative to residential provision. Secondly, the growing interest in stimulating informal networks of care and developing 'good neighbour' schemes by both social workers and organisers has demonstrated the common ground between them and shown the need for a shared approach.

Goldberg and Connelly (1982 : 254) have suggested that one way of achieving a role for organisers more compatible with the organisation of social work teams might be for them to abandon assessment functions and become home care experts within social work teams, presumably relying on social workers to carry out the assessment and review of client need. Alternatively, they felt organisers might be fully integrated into social work teams by transferring their personnel functions to administrative staff and retaining social work duties. Both these models have disadvantages. Such arrangements would require individual home helps to be responsible to two different managers – one concerned with client care and the second with financial, administrative, and personnel issues; this might entail separate staff assessing the need for a service from those making financial assessments, yet the service provided sometimes depends on the charge the client is asked to pay. Similarly, it might divide responsibility for informing home helps about their duties between officers responsible for assessing client need and those concerned with conditions of service and health and safety legislation. Integrated care between social workers and home helps is a prized objective, but the fragmented management of home helps is too high a price to pay for it.

A number of experimental schemes have been developed to provide integrated domiciliary care services. One such scheme, described by McGrath and Hadley (1981), seeks to build on informal care and formally organised voluntary support at local neighbourhood level by decentralising services and bringing them under the control of a social worker, each social worker organising the work of ancillary staff including home helps. There are undoubted benefits from such a form of organisation and some members of the Barclay working party regarded it as a prototype for the provision of social welfare services in the future, pointing out that where services are organised on this basis there is evidence of closer working relationships between agencies operating locally, higher referral rates, earlier intervention, and a greater development of voluntary initiatives.

Another experimental model which also deploys social workers as the prime co-ordinators for services entails giving them control of a budget which they allocate in order to 'buy' the services they need. Evaluation studies have found that such a system facilitates a more flexible approach to the provision of services and the imaginative use of new resources such as 'good neighbours' who perform certain tasks in return for payment.

Both these experimental models place social workers in the role of co-ordinator and 'keyworker' for a range of services. By clarifying lines of communication, they assist the mobilisation of many different services to provide care for the individual in need. They do not, however, obviate the necessity for skilful and specialist provision from the range of professionals involved.

There is scope for much more experiment in the provision of services and for careful evaluation of different organisational approaches. There is every reason to believe that, given adequate preparation and training, home helps can make a greater input than they have in the past if they work in close collaboration with other staff, and that informal carers and paid 'good neighbours' can be encouraged to provide care by sensitive and co-ordinated action. There is particular scope for an extension of special rehabilitation schemes involving regular reporting back to assist all the professionals involved to evaluate progress. A notable feature of every special scheme described in Chapters 3 and 5 is the close involvement of home helps and their first-line supervisors with specialist staff, including social workers, psychiatrists, family doctors, and psychologists.

If social workers are to manage home helps, they must familiarise themselves with employment legislation; they must undertake the necessary paperwork that accompanies the employment of staff; they must monitor performance and ensure that complaints and problems are properly handled, and that appropriate action is taken when things go wrong. As well as assessing the needs of individual clients, they will be required to assess priorities and to ration services by moving home helps from one client to another in response to changing pressures. In short, they will be expected to become home help organisers. Doubtless, some social workers would be willing to carry out these tasks, but they could only do so to the detriment of other work which hitherto they have felt to be more central to their training, experience, skill, and function.

Some of the problems facing the home help service are unique. No other social welfare service employs large numbers of manual workers with no static workplace. This poses special problems of recruitment, selection, placement, supervision, training, termination, and manpower planning. Communication and consultation with staff require special approaches under these circumstances; terms and conditions of employment and working arrangements are also discrete. Where the service is controlled by staff with wider responsibilities, these factors may not be sufficiently understood.

A home help needs the protection of an organiser whose task it is to ensure that she is working effectively within her abilities and within the law. It would be too easy for an enthusiastic professional, anxious to develop his service, to misuse a home help by placing too great a burden on her. A hospital consultant determined to discharge a patient early, a general practitioner wanting to keep a dying patient at home, a social worker trying to prevent an old person from needing a residential place or endeavouring to keep a family together to avoid the need to receive children into residential care – all have a high investment in success and may overrate the capacity of a home help and be unavailable when she needs to discuss her work. At the other extreme, they may underrate the capacity of the service and misuse an expensive resource.

In whatever specialist settings home helps operate there is a role for the home help organiser because she has a special expertise of her own based upon her knowledge of legal requirements and the capabilities of her workforce. In former years, discussion about the admission of the elderly to residential accommodation commonly took place between medical officers, social work staff, and staff representing residential services. Increasingly, it is becoming clear that the home help organiser has her own distinctive input into discussions of this kind. She has a key resource that enables the elderly frail to live at home, and may have more knowledge about the client's day-to-day capacity to cope than any other member of the caring team.

Anthea Hey has suggested (1977 : 2–5) that social welfare services can be classified into three main types of activity: first, social work, in which individuals and their families are helped to maintain and develop their capacities by counselling; secondly, specialist services, embracing the skills of mobility officers, occupational therapists, and those engaged in education and training for such groups as children and the handicapped; and thirdly, basic services which are directed towards meeting day-to-day human needs. In this latter category Hey places feeding, clothing, cleanliness, and the upkeep of accommodation. Describing the creation in 1971 of social services departments in England and Wales and the bringing together of these various functions, Miss Hey, herself a distinguished social worker, says,

'In many instances the enforced marriage was founded on a false assumption that social work was the superior partner instead of working through to achieve the potentials of both partners . . . it seems as though the social work element gets a disproportionate amount of attention. When other elements do get attention it must be very galling to the staff concerned when remedies tend to contain prescriptions to put more social work influence, knowledge, skills and attitudes into the mix.'

In another attempt to destroy the myth that the profession of social work can, does, and should control all professional activity in social services and social work departments, Cherry Rowlings says, unequivocally,

'Not every client will require or want social work support and certainly the provision of social service should not be dependent upon a social work recommendation. Nor is it feasible or even desirable that every client referred for social service also receives a separate assessment to see if social work help is appropriate.'   (1981 : 66)

This is a particularly valuable comment because it is made by an experienced social worker who has also been involved in considerable research into the operation of social services teams.

The role of a home help organiser can be very limiting if it is restricted to the assessment of need relating to the provision of a home help. There is an imbalance between the depth of understanding required to carry out the task and the range of provision available. A social worker usually has little control over resources, but is responsible for securing the most appropriate help for each of her clients, using resources controlled by her own agency and those of voluntary organisations, health, housing, education, and income maintenance services. In contrast, the responsibility of the home help organiser is generally restricted to a very narrow remit.

It is in recognition of the need to make better use of the talents and skills possessed by organisers that many authorities have extended their responsibilities to embrace the full range of basic home care services, such as meals-on-wheels, home laundry, night-sitters, and the deployment of volunteers on personal caring functions. These duties require the same assessment skills that are used to determine the need for home help provision and in many cases represent an alternative means of achieving the same objective.

The development of a more comprehensive model for the provision of home care services requires a change of nomenclature for the organiser, who then becomes accountable for a wider range of functions. Some authorities have recognised this development and changed the name of the service to the 'home care service', organisers to 'home care organisers', and home helps to 'home care assistants'. This widening of role, taken together with appropriate training and considerable management responsibility, makes it difficult to justify the fact that organisers are generally on a much lower salary scale than social workers. The number of social workers employed, their articulateness, and the proportion of university graduates involved have helped to improve salary levels in recent years. The future will no doubt see strong pressure for improving the conditions of employment of organisers and increased opportunities for them to be seconded on professional training courses.

Given an equality of status between home help organisers and field social workers, we may expect a far higher proportion of organisers to progress to senior management positions in social welfare services. In a department that develops home care services and provides professional and post-professional training, we see no reason why a home help organiser should not have equal promotion prospects with field and residential social work staff to the post of director of social services; but it is likely to be well into the twenty-first century before the first such appointment occurs.

The health service has adopted a system of functional management whereby different professional groups such as doctors, nurses, and administrators are separately accountable. Although doctors are held in great esteem they are not managerially responsible for the work of other groups of staff. A district health authority is managed by a team of officers, each representing a particular professional interest.

The strict application of this style of functional management is not possible in social welfare services as they are currently structured in Great Britain. A local authority department is headed by a chief officer who is accountable for all the work carried out in his department. It is a matter for decision in each authority how services are organised below the chief officer. As described in Chapter 4, it may be decided to have a unified home help service with a separate chain of accountability from locally based organisers to an organiser at headquarters who will work alongside other heads of services below the chief officer. On the other hand, the prime goal may be for an integration of services at more local level, in which case social work, home help, occupational therapy, residential care, and day services may be grouped under specialist managers at intermediate levels in the department, with accountability to two or more area directors. Either model will work satisfactorily depending upon the management and professional abilities of those appointed to senior positions. However, if an area structure is preferred it is important that salary gradings for home help managers are comparable to those of other managers at area level.

In the past, authorities that have developed a unified service with a centrally based manager have probably been better able to maximise the potential of the service. Experience of meeting large numbers of organisers from many parts of the country, both individually and in groups, suggests that in these authorities organisers are more likely to have high self-esteem and feel that their views are taken into account when new developments are planned. They also feel better informed about matters affecting the service. Such authorities are more likely to have well considered policies on recruitment, training, and priorities for allocating work and for developing new services.

There can, however, be no single prescription for the organisation of services which suits all authorities. Undoubtedly, the goal should be the close integration of services at local level since, in the long run, that is how barriers will be broken down and how the service can maximise its potential, developing high-calibre organisers who themselves can antici-pate promotion to broader management roles, thus further enriching and integrating services. The problem of poor integration of community care services principally arises from a lack of co-ordination between profes-sionals. As the health service has learned, this cannot be resolved by placing one group of professionals under the control of another. That way lies discontent on a large scale and friction which can jeopardise services for more than a generation.

Clients in need are entitled to expect more than an integrated programme of assessment and care from their social services department. They may require assistance from health services which suffer from equally formidable problems of co-ordination among staff based in different buildings serving a variety of geographical areas and offering different skills. Beyond this there is a need to ensure that services provided by housing authorities and voluntary organisations are com-patible and are offered to clients in a co-ordinated way.

Again, it is tempting to believe that if one professional group were made responsible for co-ordinating or controlling all domiciliary services there would be an improvement in the delivery of services, leading to a more effective use of money and manpower. Given the number of professional groups contributing their skills and judgement, it is difficult to see how one individual could weld them into an integrated team. An understanding of other professionals, how they work, and what they can achieve, is an essential part of the training and practice of all groups of staff in the caring professions. Good professional practice demands a willingness to understand and co-operate with a variety of staff; where that willingness is absent, the creation of co-ordinators is unlikely to be of value.

Many hospitals have developed administrative systems for ensuring that domiciliary services are notified of the needs of patients prior to their discharge; geriatric units have made considerable progress in this direction, although the elderly in acute hospital wards often receive an inferior service. We have already noted that some home help organisers are based in hospitals to facilitate the flow of information and ensure the prompt allocation of services when patients are discharged from hospital. There is also a need for easy contact between social services personnel and the primary health care team of general practitioner, health visitor, and community nurse. Where particularly complex problems arise a case conference may help to identify key issues and facilitate agreement about the roles of the staff concerned.

When continuing support in the home is required, the concept of 'keyworker', in which one member of staff agrees to accept prime responsibility and is contacted by other professionals if significant changes occur, can be valuable. Thus a home help organiser may be regarded as the keyworker in respect of a household and have the task of ensuring that relevant services are made available as required. This is a far better system than an unco-ordinated approach in which the general practitioner, health visitor, community nurse, social worker, occupational therapist, and home help organiser each approach the social security services, the local housing department, or voluntary agencies about the same client, unaware of the actions of other members of the team.

If organisers are to be responsible for all practical support services and assume the role of keyworker in a significant number of instances, the number of organisers will need to be increased. Furthermore, they will need increased assistance to pursue enquiries with other organisations, notably social security and housing departments. Since so much social work activity with the elderly is undertaken by welfare assistants, there would be merit in the latter working to home help organisers to provide a more comprehensive service, approaching social workers when their specialist skills were required.

The only legitimate response to the growing complexity of health and social services provision is improved co-ordination. Nostalgic references to the old-fashioned family doctor, who practised total care for his patients and commanded instant respect and obedience, do not do justice to the complex diversity of skills now available in the caring services, or to the extent to which clients with severe physical and mental problems are being supported in the community and provided with something more than basic physical care. It is not realistic to assume that social workers can replace the omnibus duties of the former family doctor. Pluralistic professional care services are here to stay.

12 · Staff training
and development

HOME HELPS

In contrast to most other countries which provide home help services there has been only a modest development of staff training schemes in the United Kingdom. The reasons for this different approach are complex and arise from a number of interrelated factors. There has been uncertainty about the aims of the service, and until there is common agreement about what is to be achieved it is not possible to identify the skills required or the training that is necessary to equip staff with those skills. In the United Kingdom there has been an almost universal assumption that the service should be provided by middle-aged women, working part-time, who have no skills to offer the labour market other than their knowledge of housework. This assumption has not been made in other European countries where there have been vigorous efforts to attract young women and to provide them with training and a career job.

During the early years of the service home helps were deployed as untrained assistants to health visitors and district nurses. It was felt that guidance from trained nurses enabled them to work satisfactorily as ancillaries, specialising in the same household tasks that would be undertaken by the home helps in their own homes. The potential for further development and a widening of this role soon became clear and, as has already been described, in the 1940s and early 1950s services expanded to embrace night-sitting, residential care, and the rehabilitation of a wide variety of client groups.

At the 1952 home help conference in Oxford a succession of speakers from European countries outlined their training schemes in detail. The

Belgian delegate described a national training programme of 200 hours followed by supervised practice for six months. The conference was informed of courses lasting six months in the Netherlands followed by a practice year. In Norway courses provided for 200 hours of academic study and 240 hours of practical experience. In France theoretical and practical training lasted seven months; in Austria eight months, Sweden fifteen months, Switzerland eighteen months, and in Finland two years.

At that time local authorities in the United Kingdom relied on the National Institute of Houseworkers to provide training for home helps. Six experimental courses commenced in 1951 lasting between twenty-seven and sixty-two hours each. Some local authorities provided their own in-service training, but this rarely exceeded a few hours. The United Kingdom delegates at the Oxford conference were stunned to learn of the wide disparity in training between the United Kingdom and other countries, and the lost potential for development; over thirty years later we have barely begun to redress the balance.

From the beginning, the relationship between the National Associ-ation of Home Help Organisers (to become the Institute of Home Help Organisers in 1954) and the National Institute of Houseworkers was strained. The latter was established in 1946 with the primary task of raising the status of domestic employment. It provided training courses of six months' duration and awarded a diploma in housecraft. The training was designed for girls and young women who were seeking residential posts in hospitals, hotels, training colleges, boarding schools, residential homes, and in private houses.

In co-operation with the London County Council arrangements were made in 1948 for ninety-two existing home helps to undertake the practical examination of the National Institute of Houseworkers; as a result eighty-one diplomas were awarded and detailed proposals were made to the county council for an eighteen-day training programme for home helps. Similar examinations were carried out in eight other local authority areas.

Home help organisers were generally critical of the training provided by the National Institute of Houseworkers. They felt the courses were designed more to meet the needs of young girls, rather than the older women who made up such a large proportion of the home help workforce. They wanted more instruction to be provided on how to approach difficult families, and specific training on the care of the aged, the housebound, the bedfast, the mentally ill, and children in need. The London County Council withdrew support from the National Institute because the courses were felt to be unrealistic.

In retrospect, the failure of the home help service to achieve a satisfactory working relationship with the National Institute of House-workers was of crucial importance, and an opportunity to make a lasting impact on the quality of provision was lost. The institute had government backing, and if it had been possible to reach agreement on a syllabus it is likely that within a few years a nationally recognised system of training could have been developed which would have done much to raise the level of the service. The failure in the 1950s to exploit the resources and facilities then available has cost the service dearly. Instead of a nationally recognised training and qualification, many local *ad hoc* schemes exist of varying scope and quality.

As a former president of the International Council of Home Help Services has said, 'to be born a female is not in itself sufficient preparation for the home help service' (National Council of Home Help Services 1976 : 7). Nevertheless, widespread doubts have been expressed about the wisdom of providing training for home helps. The belief, so commonly held, that the home help merely undertakes in other people's homes simply what she does in her own is based on an assumption that her function does not extend beyond basic household cleaning. But even if that were so, she would need to learn about the different problems of clients with a variety of disabilities. For example, she must be made aware of the need to replace furniture and other items exactly as before in the home of a blind client, and to ensure that cooking and other equipment is left in easy reach for a client in a wheelchair. She must learn to respect the foibles of the elderly, who may hoard apparently worthless personal possessions which represent for them a lifetime's treasures of great sentimental value. She must learn to cope with incontinence without undermining the pride and personal dignity of the client.

But the home help service is about more than cleaning; it is about personal relationships, about instilling a sense of purpose into the lives of people who are disabled, anxious, and depressed; it is about helping clients to achieve independence and encouraging them to undertake tasks unaided. Such functions require knowledge and skill which must be taught.

Concern is sometimes expressed that the provision of training will make home helps dissatisfied. This was recognised by the Institute of Home Help Organisers in the 1950s when it stated: 'It has been said that to give formal training to women already in possession of a background of household management, including the care of children, tends to rob them of their initiative, makes them status conscious and unwilling to undertake the less pleasant tasks or to do many of the duties assigned to them' (1958a : 20). The same kind of comment was made at a seminar in 1974 when it was said that there was 'some feeling that training might have disadvantages and that home helps were the last remaining link between neighbourliness and trained staff' (DHSS 1976 : 37).

Similar arguments were used in the nineteenth century to resist universal education, yet it was recognised that without improved education the needs of industry for a literate workforce could not be met. The answer to the problem, now as then, is not to restrict education and training but to ensure that through a variety of training schemes the workforce is able to achieve its full potential, and to structure the service so that it is possible to deploy differing skills.

Early training schemes for home helps laid great emphasis on health and hygiene. This reflects the original concern of the service to prevent the spread of infection and to improve diet and cleanliness in the home. Considerable importance was attached to economical cooking, possibly as a consequence of food shortages during the war and the early post-war period. A specimen syllabus prepared by the Institute of Home Help Organisers included a session on 'household mending, including darning socks, patching bed and table linen, wool, cotton and patterned fabric. Renovation to children's and old people's garments, "Make do and Mend".' A test for staff completing the course included cleaning and renovating a felt hat.

Society has changed considerably in the past thirty years. Living conditions have improved; basic standards, including those for the elderly and handicapped, have risen; much drudgery has been taken out of household tasks by labour-saving domestic equipment; refrigerators, deep freezers, and convenience foods have revolutionised the kitchen. The importance of these changes, together with the increased numbers of highly dependent people now living in their own homes, has significantly changed the tasks of home helps. Their primary function is no longer as household cleaners; they are first-line carers for the vulnerable.

Many home helps are themselves uncertain about the need for training and there are problems to be overcome in developing comprehensive training schemes. Staff often see themselves as essentially *practical* people and are doubtful of the relevance of formal training. Training is expensive to organise; in order to release home helps to attend courses less time must be allocated to clients or staff must be paid for additional hours; there may also be considerable travelling costs involved, together with fees for outside lecturers.

It is important to create a relaxed atmosphere on courses, recognising that formal training is something quite new to the staff concerned. On evaluation, following the basic home help course in Avon, most home helps indicate that they did not want to attend; however, most request to join one of the specialist courses that follow.

The Local Government Training Board thought in 1978 that 'on the best estimate only 15% of authorities are providing systematic training for all their new home helps' (p.3). This is a matter of concern, not least because it indicates that few staff are adequately instructed on health and safety requirements or the personal needs of clients. The home help workforce is dispersed with staff working in other people's homes with a minimum of supervision; it is important to reduce the inevitable sense of isolation that arises in such circumstances and to ensure that staff are fully aware of what is expected of them.

Basic training programmes for home helps should be geared towards meeting the needs of the large number of middle-aged women with family commitments who work part-time, since they continue to form the backbone of the service. However, the changing role of home helps and the likely employment situation in future suggests that increased efforts should be made to recruit and train young people who will make their careers in the service; they are more likely to be attracted if training is provided and there is a prospect of advancement.

The Local Government Training Board recommends a package that includes induction training for new home helps lasting twelve hours, a basic training course of twenty-one hours to be attended by all home helps during the first year of their service, and optional courses including specialist subjects ranging from three to thirty hours (1978 : 6). The Institute of Home Help Organisers recommends a similar pattern of training, although there are differences in the length of courses and their content (1975 : 6–10). For example, the institute recommends that induction training should be for one day, and that basic training should be of two kinds – initial and intermediate – each lasting from thirty-six to forty hours. The minimum training recommended by the Local Government Training Board is thirty-three hours, and by the institute, seventy-eight hours.

The syllabus used for the home care service in Avon varies from nationally recommended models. The Avon training lays greater emphasis on the needs of clients than on household management, which predominates in the Local Government Training Board syllabus. Induction training, which takes place in the first week following appointment, includes a session in which the organiser provides information about the work and departmental procedures, with assistance from a check list; there follow three days in which the new recruit works alongside an experienced home help, and three hours of visiting with a district organiser to assist home helps in their appreciation of some of the factors to be taken into account by an organiser in assessing the needs of clients. During the induction course home helps are notified of the date of the next available basic training course, which provides six half days (twenty-four hours) of seminars and lectures at a local college; this course covers such items as a description of the service and its functions, the role of the organiser, conditions of service, health and safety factors, and the effect of bereavement. Within three months of undertaking the basic course a three-hour evaluation exercise is undertaken between the home help and a senior organiser, to discuss the way in which the home help has applied her learning to her work and to identify any outstanding training needs. This evaluation exercise has proved to be a valuable means of revealing weaknesses in the recruitment and induction procedures used by the county.

Following basic training, the home help in Avon is allocated to one of five social care courses covering different aspects of client disability – the physically handicapped, the elderly frail, the mentally disordered, child care, and the blind and deaf. Each client disability course is college-based and covers six sessions lasting a total of twenty-four hours. More recently courses on mental disorder have been divided so that staff can choose to undertake the whole course, lasting a total of twenty-four hours, or modules of twelve hours, each covering either mental handicap or mental illness. Similar arrangements have been made in respect of the course for the blind and deaf. Depending on the need identified by district organisers and the interest shown by staff, a home help may, during a period of several years, undertake two or more courses in client disability. A new home help in Avon undertakes a minimum of three different courses and an evaluation exercise before being regarded as fully trained; the training extends for seventy-one hours and is usually completed in the first year of service. It can be followed by more specialist training, including courses in first aid, together with short refresher courses.

The social care training, whilst teaching practical skills, also covers physical and psychological aspects of disability, leisure activities, physiology, mobility, and institutional care. The child care course covers child abuse, legal obligations, report writing, early growth and development, and fostering and adoption; an account of court procedures is included to prepare home helps for a possible court appearance in care proceedings. First aid training, although optional, is very popular with Avon home helps, and it is clear that the skills they learn on these courses have been of immense value in their day-to-day work, particularly with children and the infirm. Advanced training is provided in Avon for home aides who offer more intensive care for the physically and mentally frail. The training includes a period of observation in physiotherapy and occupational therapy departments of a hospital, and opportunities to take part in, and observe, work in hospital wards and elderly persons' homes.

Arrangements for the training of Avon home care staff have been made in conjunction with a local technical college. Two-fifths of the salary of a college lecturer are met from the social services training budget. The lecturer, a qualified home help organiser, serves as tutor for all home help training. The use of the college means that course organisation and administration, accommodation and domestic arrangements, are undertaken by the college, and the library is available to all students. The social services department retains responsibility for the content of courses; all proposals for training are considered at management meetings of senior home help staff attended by the college lecturer.

Within the limited resources at its disposal the Local Government Training Board has prepared plans for offering practical encouragement and advice to local authorities on the training of home helps. As well as providing grants to authorities for courses designed to prepare home help organisers for training responsibilities in respect of their staff, it is proposed to offer financial support to authorities for training home helps. The scheme commenced in 1983.

If the service is to offer good career opportunities to new entrants and make use of all their potentialities, it is essential that a nationally agreed training scheme is drawn up with certificates of proficiency that are recognised for grading and promotion purposes. The training should be supervised by the Local Government Training Board and organised jointly by social services departments and local colleges. There are many different views about the style, content, and duration of training courses for home helps, and the first task will be to reach agreement between all the interested parties on a common approach, but the model adopted by Avon might be the starting-point for discussion.

As well as a number of specialist options relating to the needs of different client groups, there would be advantages in establishing courses at an advanced level and for this training to be recognised by higher pay. Certificates should be awarded to candidates based on an assessment by course tutors of both classwork and practical placements. Advanced courses would include a short written examination.

The Local Government Training Board would find it necessary to ensure that the method and content of home help training was monitored and that changes were made in the light of experience and the changing of the work. It should also advise and encourage local authorities on the provision of refresher courses and study days. Each home help should have opportunities for at least twenty-four hours of in-service training every year.

The creation of a trained workforce will not make the service easier to manage. Training encourages home helps to be more aware of the potential of the service and also of their own limitations; they will require increased time to discuss the difficulties they encounter, and are more likely to press for improvements in services to meet unmet needs; they will want to be given opportunities to contribute their views and knowledge when plans are formulated in respect of the clients they serve.

This greater sense of awareness and articulateness is not always welcomed by managers, or by other professional groups whose previous experience of home helps is that they passively do as they are told without asking questions and never openly challenge the views of social workers, doctors, and nurses. However, sensitive and skilled managers find that training greatly increases the capacity of home helps to sustain disturbed and deteriorated clients in their own homes and to do this by making maximum use of informal carers and other services. A trained and knowledgeable workforce serves as an ambassador for the social services, informing clients and the public at large of the services provided and the obstacles to extending provision; it also becomes a more reliable channel for conveying information about unmet needs to policy-makers.

HOME HELP ORGANISERS

Since its inception, the Institute of Home Help Organisers has been concerned to ensure high standards of practice and has recognised that this can only be achieved in the long term by establishing a nationally recognised qualification for organisers. A study published in 1959 showed that 69 per cent of organisers in Great Britain were over the age of 40 (Younghusband Report 1959 : 350). They came from many different backgrounds: some had previous training or experience in nursing or social work; others came from industry and commerce. They were uncertain about their role and status, firmly situated as they were within health departments and surrounded by doctors and nurses who had a long tradition of professional training. In 1974, the Pearce working party found that there had been little change in the age grouping of organisers (Pearce Report 1974 : 56).

Reports on post-war conferences reveal the ambivalence of organisers to the concept of training. At a meeting in London in 1952, Miss Nora Burr, county home help organiser for Kent, in a speech frequently quoted in later years, urged strongly that organisers must have a recognised training in order to carry out their duties satisfactorily. Her comments provoked a mixed reception from her audience of organisers and local authority members. Widespread doubts were expressed about the value of training which, it was thought, might reduce the attractiveness of the job to mature women who brought much useful experience with them when they joined the service. No systematic training was then available, apart from a one-week induction course run by the Women's Voluntary Service. In contrast, in certain European countries such as Belgium, Holland, and Germany, there was already a firm policy of appointing qualified social workers to organiser posts.

There comes a time in every emerging profession when existing practitioners see proposals for training as a threat to their status. Having learned on the job and carved out a role for the service, it is difficult for existing staff to contemplate the appointment as colleagues of growing numbers of young and relatively inexperienced recruits armed with certificates of qualification. Not only are old hands sceptical of the book learning and theories of such new staff, but in a world that places considerable status on training and qualifications they feel devalued and threatened. It took much patient argument and behind-the-scenes activity by leading members of the Institute of Home Help Organisers to establish a suitable training course for organisers and to ensure that it received wide recognition. The medical profession was uncertain about the need for training organisers. Health visitors, district nurses, mid-wives, and social workers, whilst often acknowledging the need for effective training, were far more engrossed in their own training requirements.

In the 1950s health and welfare services began to recruit trained social workers in increasing numbers, but there was widespread uncertainty about whether social welfare needed trained staff and, if it did, what kind of training was appropriate. Some medical officers of health and chief welfare officers who had learned their trade in the days of the Poor Law were not convinced that their services would be enhanced by the recruitment of trained staff. There was a widespread belief that those engaged in social welfare were constructing a pseudo-profession, and that they were apeing their medical and nursing betters in demanding training and professional status. The County Councils Association announced in 1956 that social work 'does not call for a fixed period of study embracing a definite syllabus but is undertaken after a period spent alongside another worker' (*Gazette Supplement* 1956 : 160). It was against this background of ignorance and indifference about the complexities of welfare services that the Institute of Home Help Organisers fought to set standards and to develop courses of training.

Since neither employers nor educational bodies were prepared to offer more than token support to the development of professional training, the institute proceeded with its own scheme which required only minimum co-operation from outside. After four years of deliberation, the institute's training committee published recommendations in 1958 for a correspondence course of six months' duration consisting of twelve papers dealing with various aspects of the service to be posted to candidates at fortnightly intervals (IHHO 1958c : 10). Each candidate was required to submit essays after receipt of course papers, and there was a written and *viva voce* examination at the end leading to the award of the institute's certificate. The course was implemented in 1960; two years later it was reported that one-fifth of all organisers held the certificate, and that some authorities referred to the desirability of candidates being qualified in recruitment advertisements (Hamer 1962 : 15). In the light of later surveys it is likely that the number of organisers who held certificates at that time was overstated.

Social workers were the only articulate staff group in the social welfare field outside children's departments; home help organisers and the few staff working in homes and centres tended to regard themselves as medical and nursing auxiliaries. It is not surprising, therefore, that pressure for change came from social workers and social work tutors. It would have been appropriate for the government to establish a committee to enquire into the training needs of staff in health and welfare services, but social work was seen to be the key component that distinguished social welfare from medical and nursing work. The government therefore created a working party to enquire into 'the proper field of work and the recruitment and training of social workers'. This committee, under the chairmanship of Miss Eileen Younghusband, CBE (later to become DBE), reported in 1959.

The terms of reference for the Younghusband working party did not permit it to consider the training needs of home help organisers – only the extent to which social workers might combine the role of organiser. The report described the uncertainties then current about the nature of the organiser's task. Some witnesses to the working party regarded the organiser's function as mainly administrative; others felt her function contained a substantial social work element. Both the Institute of Home Help Organisers and the working party were equivocal and even confused. The institute stressed to the working party the personnel management aspects of the organiser's work and played down the social work component. Its members were alarmed at the prospect of the working party recommending that their work should be undertaken by trained social workers; they feared that the service would be swamped by college leavers and did not believe that social work training would impart the skills they saw as essential for the task of organiser.

The working party came close to such a recommendation but was too uncertain to be specific; it felt that trained social workers with experience in personnel management 'should be eligible for appointment as home help organisers or deputies' (Younghusband Report 1959 : 202), and that in each authority there should be at least one trained social worker in such a role. In calculating training needs the working party therefore estimated that 200 trained social workers would be required for the home help service. No proposals were made for the basic training of organisers or for providing social workers with management experience that would equip them for organiser posts.

In its response to the working party's report, the Association of Municipal Corporations scorned the suggestion that home help organisers might be trained social workers: it felt that their duties were primarily administrative and that if any training was required at all it 'might be . . . in household and personnel management' (1960 : 19). Social workers showed little interest in organiser posts, which in any case have been generally poorly graded and present few career opportunities.

The early development of home help provision took place within the health service while key developments in social work took place elsewhere; organisers and social workers therefore found themselves in different camps with some mutual suspicion and even rivalry. Although they have now been together in the same departments for more than ten years they have continued to develop in isolation. As Alexander Pope said more than 200 years ago,

Tis education forms the common mind,
Just as the twig is bent the tree's inclined.

The outcome of the Younghusband working party's deliberations was the creation of a Council for Training in Social Work, and a considerable financial investment by local authorities and central government in new nationally agreed training courses for social workers arranged in educational institutions. By 1964 sixteen new training courses had been established with an annual intake of 200 students. Home help organisers were left to identify and meet their own training needs through courses designed by their institute. This imbalance in meeting the training needs of organisers and field social workers has continued to the present day.

In the early 1960s the Institute of Home Help Organisers approached the Royal Society of Health for assistance in extending the scope of its training course, but the cost proved too high. Having been spurned by employers and training bodies alike, the institute turned to the only organisation expressing an interest in the provision of training for organisers – the National and Local Government Officers' Association – the trade union with the widest membership among white-collar workers in local government. This was to develop into a fruitful partnership, and in 1966 they combined to introduce a revised correspondence course and certificate with an examination consisting of four three-hour papers. In 1970 arrangements were made for the correspondence course to be linked with local colleges, candidates attending on one day each week for three terms. Two years later Chiswick Polytechnic commenced the first two-year day release course.

Because of the constraints of time and the method of study, the syllabus concentrated on the acquisition of information and knowledge rather than the development of job-related skills. The institute wished to introduce supervised practical training, but it did not have the necessary resources to extend the course content in this way and could not rely on the support of local authorities that such a development required. Members of the institute were despairingly aware of the limitations of their course and the restrictions this inevitably placed on the recruitment of high-quality staff.

The development of home care provision following the reorganisation of social welfare services in 1971 (1969 in Scotland) led the newly created Central Council for Education and Training in Social Work and the Local Government Training Board to consider the training needs of organisers. A joint working party was established in May 1973 under the chairmanship of N. J. L. Pearce to identify their training needs and to recommend appropriate training. The working party quickly assembled the key facts. It found that 10.6 per cent of organisers in England and Wales held the institute's certificate (7 per cent in Scotland). The report concluded that this small percentage reflected the difficulties that presented organisers in studying for the certificate while carrying out a full-time job, and that even those on day release found it necessary 'to do five days' work in the four days they were not at college' (Pearce Report 1974 : 34). Between 1 per cent and 2 per cent of organisers held university degrees, but the overwhelming majority possessed no formal qualification of any kind.

The Pearce working party concluded that there should be a nationally accepted award following basic training, an award that would give organisers 'status comparable to that of holders of other professional qualifications in local government and in the social services' (Pearce Report 1974 : 51); and it felt that a significant proportion of the course programme should be devoted to supervised practical training.

Unlike the Younghusband working party fifteen years earlier which proved to be a major taking-off point for social work training, the Pearce working party was not sponsored by central government and there was no commitment to find the necessary resources to effect change; the water was in any case muddied by the creation of the Birch working party on manpower and training for the social services established by the

Department of Health and Social Security within days of the publication of the Pearce Report.

As though to demonstrate its contempt for the absence of concern about training shown by central government, local authorities, and training bodies, and to demonstrate the belief of organisers that all the current talk would lead to little or no improvement, the National Institute, together with the National and Local Government Officers' Association, went ahead in 1974 with planned changes in its training course, which was reshaped and the qualification retitled 'the Diploma in Home Help Organisation'. The range of material in the course was extended, the study period was increased to two years, and the number of examination papers rose from four to six. It still proved impossible to include practical placements, but the course now placed greater emphasis on client care and on job-related skills.

The Birch working party, when it reported in 1976, proved every bit as unsatisfactory to home help staff as they had assumed it would be. The working party's terms of reference had been 'to consider the need for trained manpower in the personal social services in the light of the present state and prospective development of those services'. It decided to exclude reference to groups of staff 'whose professional discipline is not that of social work' (Birch Report 1976 : 18), and interpreted this decision as bringing home help organisers within its remit but not home helps. Although a wide range of professional associations and educational institutions were represented on the working party, home help organisers were not included. The report recognised that organisers, along with other groups of staff carrying out supervisory duties in social services departments, had been provided with few opportunities for training, and remarked that they 'should be a key group for investment in qualifying training' (p.100). A table showing the proportions of different categories of staff who were professionally qualified omitted any reference to organisers.

Primarily, the report was about manpower and training needs in relation to social workers, and it argued throughout that a social work qualification fitted staff to assume a variety of managerial and supervisory roles over staff with other forms of training. For example, the report drew attention to the fact that much first contact work was carried out by staff who did not hold full professional qualifications, and that they needed to know when to call on the services of social workers; 'such an arrangement', the report went on, 'would of course also imply that such staff were supervised by qualified social workers' (p.75). The implications for the home help service of a policy of this kind were not presented. It could be interpreted as meaning that only a social work qualification represents a full professional training and that home helps and their organisers should work directly to social workers.

The Central Council for Education and Training in Social Work was aware of the need to rationalise the training of social welfare staff that it inherited when it was formed in 1971. The council proceeded to phase out several existing qualifications for which it had responsibility and replaced them with a new qualification, the certificate in social service (CSS). This was created to meet the needs of a number of occupational groups in social welfare other than social workers, and was introduced gradually from 1975. The CSS is based on a modular pattern including day release and some block periods of study combined with practical placements. The training includes a common unit for all students, together with a number of options that relate to the job content of particular staff. Thus a single course can provide training for staff who work in diverse settings such as day care for the mentally handicapped, residential homes for children, and the home help service. The main limiting factors are the overall cost and the need to ensure that there are sufficient numbers of students undertaking each option to justify the extensive teaching arrangements required.

CSS courses are jointly managed by employing agencies and educational institutions. Students remain in their employment during training. The courses are mainly based in further education colleges, while the majority of courses leading to the certificate of qualification in social work (CQSW) are provided in universities and polytechnics. It was hoped that the CSS training programme would grow rapidly to become the qualifying course for the majority of social services staff requiring a qualification, but owing to reductions in public expenditure during the late 1970s development was curtailed, and by 1982 the Central Council for Education and Training in Social Work indicated that the student intake was just over one-third the size of that for CQSW courses.

The CQSW programme has been regarded by CCETSW as suitable for training staff in any sector of the social welfare services. CSS training, on the other hand, is related to a narrower range of functions, depending upon the optional subjects pursued by the student. Where CSS trained staff work in field services they are mainly employed as assistants to social workers. There can be no doubt, therefore, that the CSS training leads to fewer career opportunities than the CQSW training.

CCETSW announced in 1982 that it was to review its policy in relation to qualifying courses. This provides a further opportunity to rationalise training arrangements and to create a single integrated system of training for all professional social welfare staff. Similar levels of academic ability are required for many different social welfare tasks in domiciliary, day, and residential services. The format of the CSS, embracing a modular approach and requiring a partnership between employers and training agencies, has demonstrated its value. A common core of training is required for social welfare staff whether they work in domiciliary, day, or residential services. An integrated training should help to reduce inter-professional rivalries within social welfare services and should also facilitate better understanding and co-operation between staff in different parts of the service. The opportunity should be taken to ensure that, immediately following qualification, all social services staff undertake a probationary year of supervised practice.

A system of training and examination that is seen to offer qualifications that are comparable for staff undertaking different tasks, if accompanied by a rationalisation of pay scales, is likely to modify the present tendency for career-minded staff to opt for training in field social work. Such a form of training will enable new entrants to the service from related fields to choose, after taking the common core training, options that complement the skills they have already acquired. A modular approach will enable staff who wish to switch to different types of social welfare work to undertake further units of study. Thus an employee with a qualification in field social work will be able to undertake a further module to equip himself to work as a mobility officer for the blind, an instructor for the mentally handicapped, or a home help organiser. Similarly, it will provide wider career prospects for home help organisers who, with further training, could proceed to other areas of work.

The CSS has considerable advantages over the institute's diploma as a method of training. It is validated by a nationally recognised training organisation; it provides for extended periods of supervised practical work; it ensures that students are released from their day-to-day duties so that they can concentrate on their studies; and it consists of an integrated programme of study embracing college-based lectures and seminars and study supervision provided by employing organisations. However, the CSS provides as yet no professional identity, but marks out the successful student as having achieved proficiency in an area of work which remains dominated in its upper echelons by holders of the CQSW. While this situation prevails there will continue to be a clamour for staff to be seconded on CQSW courses, and the promotion of other forms of training for social welfare staff will be blighted.

It will not be easy to achieve a unified social services training based upon the CSS model. Universities are unlikely to find it acceptable to engage in such a form of training, yet will be reluctant to abandon their current responsibilities for the training of social workers. For their part, social workers will, understandably, regard a significant transfer of responsibilities for their training from universities to polytechnics and colleges of further education as a retrograde step. Yet there is no rational explanation why social work training should be regarded as more important, or be afforded a higher status, than other forms of social services training. The location of basic training courses outside universities would leave universities free to concentrate on non-professional degree courses, on post-qualification studies, and on research.

The development of integrated training for social services staff may be some years away; meanwhile the CSS training is likely to be available for only a small number of organisers. It is therefore essential that the institute's diploma continues in existence until a new form of training is generally available. A set of examination papers for the diploma is shown in Appendix 3.

The Birch working party recommended that professional social services staff should have the equivalent of two weeks' in-service training each year (p.127) and that they should, in addition, receive three months' post-qualifying training every five years (p.128). The development of staff training, even on this modest scale, cannot be achieved unless recognition is given to the need for the appointment of relief staff who will enable those being trained to be released from their day-to-day duties.

All staff in social welfare services should have equal opportunities for training and for career progression. The quality of services will be enhanced if training can be so organised that staff move freely between different branches of the service. Future generations will find it curious that in the last quarter of the twentieth century social welfare services in the United Kingdom were integrated administratively but not professionally. That is the next important task to be tackled; not merely to improve the quality of services but to ensure that the very considerable sums spent on staff training are used to the best advantage.

13 · Directions
for change

Human existence is a story of conflict and reconciliation; of tension between States and between groups of people within States pursuing different ideals; of struggles for power and supremacy; of religious, political, and social movements aimed at changing attitudes, narrowing areas of conflict, and reconciling warring factions.

Just as the world is divided into different nations, so within each nation there are many diverse groups jostling with one another to satisfy their needs and to implant their particular vision of the truth on those around them. In poor societies, where people are mainly concerned to secure the means for basic physical survival, the principal role of government has been to protect its citizens from external attack, to preserve law and order, and to underpin the authority and power of the person or persons in control. But the creation of wealth on a large scale and its dispersal throughout society have brought demands for social justice and for governments to recognise the needs and aspirations of the disadvantaged.

Governments in modern industrial societies have found it necessary to reduce social tension and conflict by ensuring that the bulk of the population has access to services that meet basic needs for food, warmth, shelter, and medical care, and to ensure that wealth, income, and power are distributed in ways that are generally acceptable. A government that is not seen to be attempting to meet these basic human needs and aspirations will not survive. In a democracy it will be replaced through the ballot box; in a totalitarian regime it will be weakened by subversion and risk insurrection; eventually it must change or fall. State supported services in industrial societies can, therefore, be regarded as a necessary response by governments to demands of the population. They are, in themselves, a means of reducing conflict and of producing social cohesion, without which government of any kind would become impossible.

Public services cannot, of themselves, produce social harmony; they merely help to create conditions that reduce conflict. As evidenced in Northern Ireland and elsewhere, unless political power and the processes of government are seen to be responsive to the demands of the population as a whole, no amount of public services will prevent social tension. All human history demonstrates that the human spirit places social justice and personal dignity above physical comfort.

The flexible partnership between families and the State which characterises social care in western democracies is by no means a universal phenomenon of industrialised countries. In a number of eastern European countries, legal requirements are placed upon families to provide care. This applies in Poland, Hungary, and Yugoslavia. Persons who provide intensive home care for a relative in Czechoslovakia improve their own pension rights.

In western countries the individual takes his chance in an economic system that produces an uneven distribution of income and wealth but endeavours to provide a wide choice of lifestyles; in eastern Europe there is more financial security for individuals and greater uniformity, with the family having little choice about its caring role. Inevitably, the changes that have been wrought in family life during the last fifty years in the western world will gradually spread to other nations. By the turn of the century more countries will be developing home help services to meet the pressures of industrial life. An extended International Council of Home Help Services could become a major forum for identifying and discussing the impact of economic and ideological systems on family functioning.

The most serious and socially damaging problem currently facing western countries is undoubtedly the large number of people doomed to long-term unemployment. The reaction of the United Kingdom government to this problem is to provide modest work experience and training schemes and to develop ways of encouraging industrial growth, in the hope that the recession will be temporary and that in due course the economy will recover to bring full employment once again.

There are reasons to doubt whether the current economic recession will follow a cyclical pattern. Industrial and technological changes make it unlikely that many of those now unemployed will ever work again in industry, because new production techniques and even new office technology will require new skills and fewer employees. Special strategies are required to tackle the problem of large-scale and long-term unemployment. Merely to put faith in an upturn in the economy is to ignore the fundamental and rapid changes taking place in industry, and the fact that large numbers of people now unemployed will not be absorbed into jobs by an industrial revival. The crisis is not solely or even primarily about unemployed school leavers, but about the growing army of men and women with family responsibilities who face long-term unemployment.

Creating jobs that do not contribute to national wealth is unattractive at a time when any funds that can be found might be better employed by investment in industry to increase competitiveness and to create wealth, without which there can be no satisfactory solution to the country's economic problems. It is on this basis that recent governments have sought to reduce public expenditure and urged local authorities to shed staff. The economic logic behind this approach is impeccable and might even be attractive if there were no social consequences, but the social effects of unemployment are a good deal more severe than is generally recognised and, in themselves, create additional public expenditure. Unemployment is costly in financial terms and it represents an under-use of the most valuable resource available – the human spirit; economic recovery cannot be bought by squandering the nation's chief asset.

Despite reductions in public expenditure in recent years, considerable sums are still spent and will always be spent on social care for the sick, the elderly, and other groups such as delinquents. Nevertheless, services for these groups are starved of funds, and although there are agreed strategies promulgated by central government for making improvements, these remain unfulfilled ambitions because the resources are simply not being made available to implement desirable change.

Ironically, the kind of labour needed to transform social care is precisely that which now forms a huge percentage of the unemployed and which, under present policies, is likely to remain unemployed for the foreseeable future. Many of the basic services needed to care for people in their own homes require modest skills and training, well within the capabilities of large numbers of the unemployed. Home help provision, day care, night-sitting services, and short-term fostering for dependent groups such as the handicapped and the elderly, are vital ingredients in providing effective services enabling people in need to stay in their own homes, yet they do not necessarily require highly developed and scarce skills. Personal integrity, self awareness, a capacity to relate to people in difficulty, and a willingness to help others are all attributes to be found in abundance among the unemployed; with modest training, a marginal increase in management costs, and little extra in the way of equipment, they could be provided with worthwhile work. A plentiful supply of managers can be found from the ranks of graduates who are unemployed or employed in jobs that do not make full use of their talents.

The country must be prepared to accept the social consequences of industrial change and face the challenge that it brings. If ways can be found of curbing inflation while at the same time deploying a larger proportion of the workforce on socially desirable activities, the quality of life will be enhanced for us all. New technology will bring increased leisure, but it will also bring disillusionment, frustration, and social disintegration unless it gives a meaning to people's lives. The degradation of large-scale and long-term unemployment can be replaced by absorbing, worthwhile, and creative work if acceptable ways are found to share equitably the fruits of modern technology. Central government must take the lead in bringing this about.

The development of services for disadvantaged groups raises expectations among them for better services and encourages them to press for further improvements. Following the Chronically Sick and Disabled Persons Act of 1970 which greatly extended the entitlement of handicapped persons to services from local authorities in England and Wales, not only did services expand dramatically but the strident and critical view of the consumer became audible. By conferring rights and raising levels of service, legislation revealed hidden needs which were articulated for the first time. Experience suggests that as services expand so public criticism about the quality and quantity of provision increases; indeed, an authority with highly developed services sometimes receives more public complaints than a neighbouring authority which provides a lower level of service.

As disadvantaged groups in society become less disadvantaged, so their power to influence public policy increases. When the handicapped have mobility allowances and facilities that enable them to lead more normal lives, they become visible and can more easily press for further improvements. Rising numbers of elderly and handicapped people in the population lead them to wield considerable voting power which cannot be ignored; they are also more articulate about their needs than former generations. Improved financial benefits for the elderly and handicapped and the growing number of occupational pension schemes mean that they are a very important consumer group: it has been estimated that the oldest 20 per cent of the United States population account for 27 per cent of all consumer spending. This is an indication of the changing distribution of power in modern society which is likely to accelerate in all western countries leading to increased demands for higher quality social welfare services.

In the United Kingdom, as in many other western countries, there is a widespread belief that essential health and social welfare services should be provided by the State and be provided free of charge to consumers, or carry a heavy public subsidy. This is in contrast to other countries, notably the United States, where provision through voluntary and private agencies is the norm and where private insurance is encouraged as a means of meeting costs.

The increasing cost of modern medical technology, the rising demand for health care, and the desire for lower tax levels are pushing governments into exploring alternative ways of financing public services. The British government has been examining how health services might be financed by private insurance and, as increasing numbers of elderly people become eligible for earnings-related state pensions together with occupational pensions, it will become progressively more attractive to seek ways in which the users of services increase their contribution towards the cost. It can be argued that the first priority of governments should be to ensure that the elderly and others in need receive an adequate income so that they can exercise choice in the use of services. For these reasons the movement in the early 1970s for free home help services in England and Wales did not gain momentum, and it is likely to be overtaken in the next decade by a policy of increased charges. Care will be required to ensure that, as charges rise, adequate protection is afforded to those on low incomes, and that the cumulative effect of mounting charges for a variety of services does not bear too heavily on individual clients.

By ensuring that supplementary benefit is no longer payable towards the cost of local authority home help services in Great Britain, the Social Security Act of 1980 may encourage the growth of private agencies to meet home care needs. As local authorities sharpen their charging policies and seek to recover an increasing proportion of their costs, the stage may be reached when voluntary organisations or private companies can compete on equal terms because their services will attract supplementary benefit payments. If private health insurance expands, and if a way can be found to include home care within its benefits, there could be a mushrooming of voluntary and private agencies in this field by the end of the century. A major United Kingdom organisation providing medical insurance has indicated to us in a private communication that it does not anticipate diversifying its benefits to include the provision of home care services. It says that research has shown that the majority of people want a low-cost insurance scheme to help towards the cost of private accommodation and treatment in the acute phase of an illness, and doubts whether the introduction of a benefit for home care provision would reduce the length of hospital stay. This situation may change.

Many arguments about the privatisation of home helps appear to rest on the assumption that they carry out a cleaning service which, subject to suitable arrangements about the provision of financial subsidies, could be carried out equally well by private agencies. The role now being carried out by a large number of home helps extends well beyond household cleaning. Whilst the work could be carried out by profit-making organisations, it would be difficult for public bodies to monitor performance and would have the effect of inhibiting the full development of the service. The use of voluntary organisations, whilst open to similar objections, does not present such serious obstacles.

The fact that the Committee of Ministers from the Council of Europe adopted a resolution about home help services in December 1977 demonstrates the international recognition given to the service. Governments of member states are recommended in the resolution to:

(1) foster and develop home help services, that is, services having a social nature and purpose, the aim of which is to provide families, or persons on their own, who are sick or in difficulty, with the help of a properly supervised, adequately trained person in the home in order to ensure the smooth functioning of the household;

(2) take account of the important role which home help services play in enabling single persons or couples who are old, sick or handicapped to stay in their homes, in avoiding or shortening institutional care for one or more members of a family in the event of illness or temporary difficulty, or in assisting either of the parents in carrying out their family and educational tasks when they are confronted with particularly acute problems.

The resolution goes on to stress the need for close collaboration between all groups in the caring professions, for good basic training, and effective organisation and research. Governments wishing to give some practical effect to the international recognition extended to the home help service by the adoption of this resolution could perhaps begin by ensuring that senior home help staff are encouraged to attend international seminars and conferences. Many United Kingdom delegates to these events meet their own expenses and some must take annual leave to attend; yet international gatherings offer an unparalleled learning experience.

The United Kingdom suffers through being an offshore island; there is a psychological barrier about using public funds to pay for delegates to attend meetings across the English Channel, yet the distances involved are sometimes little different from journeys within the United Kingdom. The sheer geographical size of countries like the United States, Canada, Australia, and even Sweden means that public bodies frequently send their staff great distances to attend meetings and conferences; on the mainland of Europe travel between countries to attend international gatherings is commonplace. The United Kingdom led the way in creating and developing the International Council of Home Help Services because key individuals were prepared to make huge personal sacrifices to improve the service in which they worked; when it comes to meeting the cost of participation in international forums, public authorities in the United Kingdom are unique in their insularity.

THE EMERGING PROFESSION

Social welfare as a concept is difficult to define, and as a consequence there have been problems in reaching agreement about who should carry it out and what skills are required by those who engage in it. Unlike education, medicine, and nursing, which carved out their roles and purpose in virgin territory, social welfare as an organised activity came late upon the scene and has pieced together an agenda from the gaps in services created by others. Those engaged in it are, therefore, aware of the need for co-operative effort and that their role must vary as other services develop and change.

But like any residual legatee, social welfare has inherited a mixed bag. On the one hand its role is to maximise opportunities for choice and independence so that clients can gain control over their own lives, but it is also expected to control and contain. For example, it has a duty to protect the mentally disordered, to prevent child abuse, and to avoid neglect among old people; such tasks cannot be accomplished without exercising direct supervision over people's lives. A common feature in all social welfare work is that it seeks to create an atmosphere in which disadvantaged clients can achieve personal fulfilment, and undertakes this in surroundings which are as near to normal as can reasonably be arranged.

The low status usually afforded to domestic work has tarnished the image of the home help service and placed it in a subordinate position among the helping professions. This has led some organisers to believe that improvements in pay, conditions, and recognition will only be brought about by shifting the balance away from domestic work and towards a more personal caring role. There can be no doubt that the service in many western countries is not using its potential to the full and could greatly develop personal caring functions; however, this can only be achieved successfully if it is carried out in co-operation with nursing services, and provided home helps retain a capacity and a willingness to continue undertaking the basic domestic functions that now characterise much of their work and that will not be performed by any other service.

Those employed in home help services are aware that although their work is held in high esteem its status is very low. Staff may have felt flattered when hospital consultants, general practitioners, nurses, and social workers have said kind things about them and praised their dedication, but this has been in the context of the low status, pay, career prospects, and training of staff. While the service is prepared to undertake unpleasant duties that others are unwilling to perform and at the same time accept a low status, it holds no threat for other professional groups.

However, a strong, well-organised, and trained workforce, clear in its objectives and demanding an input into decision-making processes, is a new phenomenon which is beginning to emerge in some local authorities; where this has happened it has upset the traditional pecking order of the caring professions and has met with fierce resistance. At a case discussion about the admission of an elderly client to residential care, an organiser will not endear herself to other members of the team if she questions their decisions. 'Leave it to the professionals' was the patronising reply given to one organiser who queried why an old lady could not be cared for at home. Whilst teamwork is universally eulogised as leading to collaboration, it is also competitive. Successful teamwork requires mutual understanding and a respect for the skills and abilities of other members of the team. Demarcation disputes and group rivalries are as common in the personal health and social services as they are in shipyards; such disputes invariably diminish client care.

Confronted by an enormous demand for the service and a lack of central direction, organisers have generally concentrated on stretching their resources as far as possible by attempting to respond to all needs. They have not been articulate about the unmet needs of their clients and have left political and industrial agitation to others. Consequently they have not made demands on their managers or other professionals but have set up the expectation that they will continue to deal with the work allocated to them by other people without question or complaint. They have not been encouraged to make demands for their service or to argue their case effectively. They have tended not to discuss their operational problems with senior staff, who in turn, subject to greater pressures from more demanding and sophisticated groups of staff, have until recently generally failed to recognise the necessity to examine the needs and problems of the service in any depth.

Home help organisers, unlike doctors, nurses, and social workers, are frequently selected and appointed by interviewing panels with no appropriate professional advice. It would be a welcome recognition of their distinctive function if local authorities ensured that at least one organiser was a member or assessor on each such interviewing panel.

Some success has been achieved in developing distinct types of service to meet particular needs; this enables recruitment, selection, training, and supervision to be organised specifically in respect of the service being provided. There are dangers in this approach for it can lead to conflict between two distinct groups of staff. Some agencies have reported that a two-tier system often means that the lowest graded staff are allocated to clients simply because there are insufficient staff available on higher grades (Davis 1977 : 6). In these circumstances, a two-tier system becomes a way of depressing the status and earning capacity of home helps.

Nevertheless, the range of work available makes it necessary to develop more than one type of home help service. At one end of the scale is a heavy cleaning service; at the other end is a rehabilitation service for a mentally ill mother. The level of skill and training, the ability to communicate, to conceptualise about what is happening, to record and know when to report changes that occur, are significantly different between the various kinds of service provided. They will attract different kinds of recruit and offer different job satisfactions.

The deployment of a special cadre of home helps who are trained and experienced in a range of rehabilitative techniques for the handicapped, and who can help parents develop their own household and child-rearing skills, will enhance the image of the service and demonstrate its adaptability and capacity to respond to social needs that are not adequately met by any other group of staff. By linking staff training with that for other groups of local authority staff – for example, those in homes for the elderly and wardens of sheltered accommodation – it should be possible to facilitate a flow of employees between different but related services, thus enabling local authorities to offer more attractive career opportunities and creating a greater understanding among different staff.

In the United Kingdom, because the training of home helps has largely been left to *ad hoc* local arrangements, there has been no serious attempt to clarify the nature of the service and to develop a two-tier structure across the country. Many local authorities have created their own specialist schemes using many different salary scales and offering training of varying kinds. There is a need to standardise basic training courses for home helps, recognising that more than one type of training is necessary, and to establish the kind of two-tier structure for pay and conditions that has been a feature of the service in some western countries for many years.

The value of a well-trained workforce that upholds professional standards and enforces its own codes of conduct has been long recognised in the medical and nursing professions. Indeed, there is statutory backing to the General Medical Council and the General Nursing Councils. Social workers are seeking to achieve similar arrangements. At this stage in the development of the home help service it is premature to argue for a statutory system, but it is important that consideration is given to standards of conduct and that nationally approved ratios of organisers to home helps are recommended to employing organisations.

Because the service is an alternative to informal care by relatives, friends, and neighbours, organisers must collaborate with families and informal volunteers. Shorter working hours for the population generally and long-term unemployment make it likely that needs will continue to be met in this way. Encouragement, supervision, and, in some cases, the payment of expenses and small honorariums will ensure that a partnership continues between the service and the wider community in which it operates.

The part-time employment of large numbers of women in the home help workforce creates considerable management problems. Except where there is a shortage of recruits or of particular skills, there would be advantages in restricting new appointments to a minimum of twenty-seven or thirty hours a week. This would reduce the span of control for organisers, relieve the pressure on training courses, and, almost certainly, reduce staff turnover, leading to a higher quality of provision.

THE WORKING CONDITIONS OF HOME HELPS

The hard physical effort involved in housework and the emotional stress of being the principal support for very frail and dependent clients place a considerable strain on home helps. They do not have ready access to their organiser – except by telephone – and they often work in isolation for long periods. Unlike other staff, they do not have the benefit of a comprehensive training to give them confidence, and they do not enjoy the opportunities for mutual support that are derived from working as part of a group such as nurses and social workers. Home helps have fewer opportunities for advice, consultation, and supervision than any other domiciliary staff in health and social services organisations. Thus the most unsophisticated staff, with the least training and the lowest pay, carry out their duties with little support and guidance.

The fact that most home helps derive great pleasure from their work should not deceive observers into believing that there are no problems. We have seen how long hours, poor working conditions, arduous and stressful work with the physically and mentally frail, and unimaginative management have combined to produce scandalous conditions for patients in long-stay hospitals. The personal stress on the carer of attempting to meet the physical and personal needs of frail clients with insufficient resources should not be underestimated. That so many home helps undertake additional work in their own time is not only a measure of their dedication and concern: it is an indication of the pressure under which they work, and of the personal tensions and conflicts that arise when a home help accepts responsibility for the care of a client whose needs simply cannot be met by the allocation each week of a few hours of service. Care must be total: home helps know that unless they light the fire on Saturday the client will spend the day in an unheated room; unless they take the laundry home it will remain unwashed. These tasks are not their responsibility, but whose responsibility are they when needs and resources are so poorly matched?

By being asked to respond to the needs of clients, home helps inevitably accept a personal challenge and find themselves meeting as many outstanding needs as they can. They represent the expression of society's conscience; exposed to the miseries and privations of their clients, they feel they have little option but to respond as they would if they were dealing with members of their own family. As a consequence, home helps react to the deterioration or death of a client as they would if it occurred in their own family. The client's burden becomes their own, and their contract of employment relating to hours of work and rates of pay becomes a passport to an unwritten contract with the client, an open-ended commitment which says, 'I will not abandon you; I will make your life as comfortable as I can and my reward will be the satisfaction that I have done my best'. Such a commitment is unavoidable in a service that hinges on personal relationships between the carer and the cared-for, but it is only acceptable if just rewards are offered for the flexibility, skill, and sheer hard work involved.

Sometimes it is necessary for an organiser to transfer a home help from a client if it appears that the personal impact of providing care is creating an over-involvement. Perceptive organisers try to allocate work in such a way that home helps who have a tendency to over-identify with clients are moved fairly frequently. Some special schemes have recognised the personal stresses that are produced in home helps and arrangements are made to ensure that stressful work is interspersed with less demanding activity.

In their training, organisers need to develop skills in detecting when home helps need support and guidance to avoid over-involvement, but the prime requirement is for adequate time for organisers and their staff to consider such issues and a working environment that facilitates private discussion. The Stockholm system of domestic help bureaux described in Chapter 5 represents a cost-effective way of reducing isolation among home helps and encouraging informal contact with organisers. The minimum requirement is for a room in which staff can meet and relax, together with facilities for them to wash, shower, and change their clothes; additionally, a private room is necessary for discussions between individual home helps and the organiser. A base of this kind may make a convenient location for the provision of staff training and for meeting staff representing other services. Where the service operates a special scheme for neglectful mothers or other client groups in association with social workers, a bureau would serve as a base for consultation and supervision. It may also serve as a reception point for clients or their relatives seeking assistance, and for the storage of cleaning materials.

Some district social work offices or health centres have sufficient space to enable developments of this kind to take place, but day centres for the elderly and even residential homes sometimes have spare capacity. Unused community facilities in blocks of flats or sheltered housing developments may be pressed into use. The growing tendency for staff in residential homes to live elsewhere has released much staff accommodation, some of which could be converted to create home help bureaux serving the local community. The additional cost of such provision will not be great but it is important that developments of this kind are given priority when accommodation is found.

It is inevitable, however, that greater opportunities for improving the management of the service will lead to demands for lower workloads for home helps and organisers. In particular, it will be seen as manifestly unjust that home helps should be expected to attend staff meetings and come to training and supervision sessions in their own time and at their own expense.

Younger and career-orientated women are more likely in future to anticipate – and even demand – appropriate training. They will expect to be provided with labour-saving implements and the means to convey them between clients. In households where clients are bedridden they will expect equipment to be available for lifting, and they will anticipate regular discussions with social workers, doctors, and nurses about the progress of clients. In return, they will demand a level of pay commensurate with the tasks undertaken. They will see no reason why machine-minding should be more profitable than caring for people, and will be less averse than their predecessors to press for better pay and conditions.

The growth in the female workforce, particularly of married women, in the past forty years has been accompanied by strident demands that they should have the same career opportunities as men. Yet many of them need to divide their time between the roles of mother, wife, and breadwinner, they tend to change jobs more often than men, have breaks in service, and are more likely than men to seek part-time employment. All these factors make it difficult for them to secure the levels of pay and promotion opportunities that are available to their male colleagues.

Public images are difficult to change. There appears to be an almost instinctive human need to believe that those who provide a personal caring service to the needy should be hardworking dedicated individuals with no personal ambitions, no wish for self advancement, and with a saintlike contentment to remain forever on the lowest salary levels. The Equal Pay Act and other legislation designed to promote equal opportunities for women have not succeeded in changing the public image of the service. This situation could be changed very quickly by the recruitment of large numbers of male home helps, who tend to be more concerned with basic matters like pay and conditions and whose claims for more recognition, better training, improved pay, and higher status will be acceded to more readily. Current and predicted unemployment levels among men may lead to a radical change in the home help workforce in future years, but the development of the service is likely to follow closely whatever general trend emerges in society with regard to the status of women, women's employment, and their pay.

DIRECTION FROM THE CENTRE

Bearing in mind the size of the home help workforce and the level of public expenditure involved, it is a matter of continuing surprise and regret that, except in Northern Ireland, the service in the United Kingdom is not given firmer direction, advice, and encouragement from central government. There is no officer in the Department of Health and Social Security with direct experience of employment within the home help service, and there is no effective mechanism for monitoring and recording what is happening in the field. In 1981, government interest in the service reached a low ebb when it was decided that the Department of Health and Social Security would no longer collect and publish information from local authorities about the number of home helps employed and the number of households assisted. Thankfully, after pressure from various sources, this decision was subsequently reversed.

The National Council of Home Help Services is an *ad hoc* organisation providing a forum for discussing issues affecting the home help service. It has no paid staff, and is not represented on the local authority associations that help to formulate overall local authority policies and have influence over central government. The Institute of Home Help Organisers, which represents organising staff employed in the service, is seriously underfunded; it conducts its business with no financial assistance from local or central government. The institute's council members meet at weekends, largely paying their own travelling and accommodation expenses.

The service is a matter of peripheral concern to a number of organisations but central only to the National Council and the National Institute. Staff of the Department of Health and Social Security Social Work Service and their counterparts in other parts of the United Kingdom retain an interest in home help provision alongside concerns for other activities of local authorities. The Local Government Training Board and the Central Council for Education and Training in Social Work have displayed an interest in the service, but until very recently have been more engrossed in the training of other categories of staff.

There is a clear need for a national organisation in the United Kingdom with responsibility for collecting information, monitoring provision, stimulating research studies, disseminating ideas about good practice, developing training schemes, and providing advice to local authorities about the organisation and development of home help services. Such a central body would require public funding, and if there were a strong commitment among local authorities the existing National Council of Home Help Services could be expanded.

The abolition by the present government of the Personal Social Services Council in 1980 and the Children's Committee in 1981 demonstrates the improbability of it establishing and funding a new and separate national advisory body for the home help service. A freestanding organisation, committed exclusively to the needs of the service, would soon become a pressure group competing with every other interest in local government, and would become a source of embarrassment to central government and local authorities alike.

The service is so far behind in terms of staff training, salaries, and status that any public body interested in investing funds to set up a national organisation would be deterred by the realisation that a successful organisation would seek to achieve a significant increase in public expenditure to bring the service up to a reasonable standard. This is the biggest single obstacle to achieving a strong national organisation, for neither central government nor the local authority associations will willingly make the necessary investment, since they are fully aware of the deficiencies that a well-organised pressure group would urge them to overcome.

It may be feasible for the government to stimulate an existing organisation, such as the National Institute for Social Work, to focus some resources and expertise on the needs and problems of the service, although this would not be possible without additional funding. The allocation of modest government funds to the National Institute for Social Work with matching local authority support might prove the most cost-effective way of promoting a central body to stimulate ideas about the role and development of the service. This would entail a change of title for the National Institute but such a course is long overdue. Some funding might be achieved for an initial period by one or more charitable trusts meeting a share of the cost. The total sum required would not be great in relation to overall home help expenditure. For a cost representing 30p per £1000 now spent on the service it would be possible to engage five professional staff with administrative and clerical support.

A national organisation or development group within an existing organisation, bringing together representatives of local authorities, staff in related services, and training interests, together with modest staff resources, would provide a much needed focus for initiating and disseminating ideas about services in the United Kingdom. It would have the capacity to collect and interpret information about the service; it could identify good practice, advise local authorities on operational policies, promote research into organisational and financial issues, and help to ensure that new projects were evaluated. One of its key functions would be to keep managers at local level informed of developments elsewhere; it is common to find local authorities experimenting with new forms of service, the staff concerned being totally unaware that other authorities attempted to provide the same kind of service and made the same mistakes many years earlier. There is now an extensive international literature about the home help service which has made little impact on the thoughts of those directing services in the United Kingdom.

Literature about the home help service abounds with criticism of the way in which it is managed. Critics frequently censure central government for failing to offer clear guidance to local authorities, but even the severest critics seldom indicate what guidance should be offered. In truth, unless information and ideas about needs and services are brought together for analysis, and different approaches are tested by carefully controlled experiment, there is no reason to believe that advice from central government will embrace the kind of wisdom required to improve policies and practice at local level.

The proposed new organisation would work with the Department of Health and Social Security, other government departments, and training organisations to foster basic training courses for home helps and organisers and to ensure that they are nationally recognised. It would advise on post-qualification training and develop training courses for senior managers. The organisation would stimulate discussion about the role and function of the service and the different models of organisation that can be adopted to achieve different objectives. One of its early tasks would be to prepare attractive literature to ensure that information about the service is available in schools and at careers conventions. The service will not secure for itself a modern and forward-looking image unless a way can be found to build that image by way of careful publicity.

There is often popular support for the expansion of public services like education, health, and social welfare, although there may be considerable public resistance about meeting the cost involved. On the other hand, it is usually staff themselves who press for improvements in training arrangements and in organisational methods. The home help workforce has been less articulate than many others in the public service and, as a consequence, despite a massive expansion in provision during the past ten years, the quality of the service has changed very little. In the next decade, better value for money might be obtained by using additional funds, not to extend the service still further, but to improve training arrangements and to strengthen management structures.

Appendix 1
The home help
service in the
United Kingdom

year	no. of home helps			no. of organisers WTE	no. of cases	% cases over 65 years
	full time	part time	WTE			
(a) *England*						
1948[1]	3,100	8,300	—	—	58,600	—
1954[1]	3,000	30,400	—	—	215,800	62.4[2]
1960[1]	2,500	46,800	20,800	617	312,000	74.8[2]
1966[1]	2,981	61,395	30,244	878	419,000	78.6
1970	—	—	29,700	983	443,200	84.2
1971	—	—	31,500	1,058	458,600	84.7
1972	—	—	35,200	1,197	473,900	85.3
1973	—	—	38,095	1,354	524,000	85.6
1974	3,910	81,437	40,810	1,507[3]	565,300	88.1
1975	3,640	85,089	42,495	1,681	615,000	86.7
1976	3,016	85,049	42,141	1,751	652,800	87.4
1977	3,237	85,613	42,907	1,870	665,200	87.9
1978	3,457	86,779	44,693	1,974	692,900	88.3
1979	3,931	86,264	44,660	2,053	730,300	88.3
1980	4,373	86,213	46,637	2,172	743,500	88.7
(b) *Scotland*						
1979	1,327	18,457	9,487	261	57,852	90.1
1980	1,442	18,714	9,687	342	60,703	90.7
1981	1,028	18,523	9,126	350	62,749	90.8

year	no. of home helps			no. of organisers WTE	no. of cases	% cases over 65 years
	full time	part time	WTE			
(c) *Wales*						
1979			2,831	83	42,237	88.5
1980			2,959	85	44,436	87.7
1981			3,102	95	45,441	88.2
(d) *Northern Ireland*						
1978			3,156	not known	20,827	86.0
1979			3,189	not known	23,308	84.0
1980			3,076	not known	22,476	82.5
(e) *United Kingdom – total*						
1980	5,850 approx.	121,125 approx.	62,359	2,599	871,115	88.6

Notes: 1 Figures for the years 1948–66 include Wales.

2 These figures include the 'chronic sick'.

3 From 1974 onwards assistant and trainee organisers are included.

This table does not include staff in specialist schemes.

Appendix 2

Duties appropriate to home helps

1 *Household tasks*
   (a) Undertaking routine/regular household cleaning.
   (b) Preparing and cooking food.
   (c) Washing up.
   (d) Lighting fire and bringing in fuel.
   (e) Making beds.
   (f) Washing and ironing personal clothing.
   (g) Arranging for the laundering of bed linens and towels.
   (h) Shopping.
   (i) Emptying commode.

2 *Personal care*
   (a) Caring for children.
   (b) Helping with washing and bathing.
   (c) Helping with dressing.
   (d) Helping with shaving and hairdressing.
   (e) Helping with personal hygiene and toiletting.
   (f) Encouraging the use of aids provided.
   (g) Encouraging the continuation with any exercises prescribed.
   (h) Encouraging the continuation with any medication or treatment prescribed.
   (i) Supervising medicines.

3 *Social care*
   (a) Collecting pension.

(b) Collecting prescriptions.
(c) Posting and writing letters.
(d) Paying rent and other accounts.
(e) Keeping in touch with relatives.
(f) Encouraging the continuation with any hobby or social activity.
(g) Contacting GP.
(h) Making telephone calls.
(i) Helping with budgeting.

4 *Training role*
    (a) Helping families with problems to achieve better housekeeping and child care standards.
    (b) Helping elderly and disabled persons to regain and/or maintain the ability for self care.

Source: Reproduced from *The Needs of Clients and the Role and Responsibilities of Home Helps*, published by the Central Personal Social Services Advisory Committee, August 1976, by kind permission of the Department of Health and Social Services, Northern Ireland.

Appendix 3

Institute of
Home Help Organisers
Diploma Examination
1982

LOCAL AUTHORITY ADMINISTRATION

Monday, 14 June 1982
9.30 a.m. to 12.30 p.m.

Answer FOUR questions
All questions carry equal marks   *Time allowed: 3 hours*

1 Explain the structure of local government in England. Why is a distinction made between metropolitan and non-metropolitan areas?
2 In what ways do local political parties influence the working of local authorities?
3 'Despite the recommendations of the Maud and Bains Committees, local authorities generally have too many committees.' Discuss this assertion.
4 Explain the role of the chief executive of a local authority.
5 Why is there so much emphasis in local government on professional or specialist qualifications?
6 Outline the composition and functions of the National Joint Council for Local Authorities' Administrative, Professional, Technical and Clerical Services, and comment on its importance in the local government service.

7 Describe the procedure for the (external) audit of the accounts of local authorities.

8 Briefly explain the main features of the rating system, and comment on its major defects.

9 What is the doctrine of *ultra vires* and what is its significance in local authority administration?

10 How important is 'public relations' in local government, and in relation to the home help service in particular?

CLIENT CARE

Monday, 14 June 1982
2.00 p.m. to 5.00 p.m.

Answer Question 1, which is compulsory, and THREE other questions
Question 1 carries 40 per cent of the marks
All other questions carry equal marks　　　　　　　*Time allowed: 3 hours*

1 *Compulsory question*
　You receive a request from a hospital-based social worker to discuss how best to help a client being discharged in the following situation:

　Two sisters, both over 80, living alone in a large inner-city house, have had an enforced separation. The younger had major surgery and is ready for discharge, and the elder, frail and registered blind, is temporarily in a residential home following emergency admission at the time of the younger sister's hospitalisation. The blind sister has apparently enjoyed aspects of the experience away from the somewhat anxious and over-bearing sister.

　(i) State what information you would need in order to make your assessment to enable both women to return home.
　(ii) Discuss what factors the home help organiser would need to consider in the long term of this case.
　(iii) Detail briefly your expectations of the home help expected to help these clients.

2 You are asked to arrange home help support to a family with a 40-year-old mother, who has an 8-week-old mongol child, following her hospitalisation for acute depression. The husband is a long-distance lorry driver. What is your response?

3 Giving case examples from your area, discuss the involvement you have with three voluntary agencies on behalf of your clients.

4 Identify the main problems to be considered when arranging help for clients who are:
　(i) diabetic;

    (ii) suffering from pulmonary tuberculosis;
    (iii) suffering from Parkinson's disease.

5 What help would you be able to provide for a 35-year-old man, whose wife has left him to look after three children, 6, 5, and 2? What briefing would you give your home help?

6 You are asked to give a talk to a group of new home helps on 'Attitudes and relationships with clients'. Detail the points you would cover.

7 An Asian mother with poor command of English has been referred for home help service following the birth of her third child. The husband is temporarily out of the country and there are two other pre-school children. How would you select and support a home help involved in this case?

8 If resources were available, how would you best provide care for a retired nurse who has terminal cancer and is now practically bedfast. She wishes to remain in her own home.

9 A home help has reported increasing difficulty in obtaining access to an 85-year-old in a basement flat. She was originally referred by her GP. The client has become more withdrawn and the home help feels she is becoming a fire hazard. How would you advise the home help and with whom would you, as an organiser, liaise in the client's interest?

10 Comment on the following:
    (i) Clients often become unjustifiably angry/accusatory to the home help.
    (ii) Many home helps do more for their clients than is required on their job description.

ORGANISATION OF THE HOME HELP AND OTHER DOMICILIARY SERVICES I: SYSTEMS AND PROCEDURES

Wednesday, 16 June 1982
9.30 a.m. to 12.30 p.m.

Answer FOUR questions
All questions carry equal marks   *Time allowed: 3 hours*

1 How would you explain the essential nature of managerial work? Discuss the extent to which principles of management can be applied in the home help service.

2 Define the need for control over administrative functions. Select an administrative procedure of your choice and explain what steps you would take to check that the procedure is operating effectively and with the minimum of errors.

3 As home help organiser, how would you attempt to maintain effective communications with staff responsible to you? Give specific examples in support of your answer.

4 What do you understand by the system of budgetary control and what are its main features? Give examples of the application of budgetary control within the home help service.

5 You have been asked to consider the possible introduction of flexible working hours for manual staff within the home help service. Draft a *short report* for your committee setting out the advantages, the disadvantages, and limitations of flexible working hours, and how such a system might operate.

6 Discuss critically the effectiveness of relationships between the home help service and other statutory agencies. What positive steps would you advise in order to improve these relationships?

7 Explain fully what the function of the office should be to support the work of the home help organiser. Give specific examples showing the range of office services provided.

8 As home help organiser, prepare a set of notes for a talk to new members of staff in the social services department on the policy objectives, tasks, and methods of working of the home help service.

9 How can the contribution of modern management techniques assist the home help organiser in providing an effective service to clients? Give examples to illustrate your answer.

ORGANISATION OF THE HOME HELP SERVICE II: PROFESSIONAL PRACTICE

Wednesday, 16 June 1982
2.00 p.m. to 5.00 p.m.

Answer Question 1, which is compulsory, and THREE other questions
Question 1 carries 40 per cent of the marks
All other questions carry equal marks   *Time allowed: 3 hours*

1 *Compulsory question*
Charging policies vary considerably between local authorities in relation to the home help service. Discuss. Describe fully the statutory implications involved before any charges for the service can be introduced. Give three examples of current practice used by local authorities in relation to charging for the home help service.

2 Describe fully the effects of two of the following as they relate to the home help service:
   (a) arbitration and disputes procedure;
   (b) Section 13(i) of the Health Services and Public Health Act of 1968;

(c) Chronically Sick and Disabled Persons Act of 1970.
3 Following repeated requests from the trades unions for improved 'conditions of service' for home helps, the Social Services Committee has asked for a full report setting out the various improvements being sought. Prepare a report in this connection with a supporting cost statement.
4 Your authority is actively considering the introduction of a scheme to provide work experience for unemployed school leavers. Describe fully how the home help service might be included in such a venture.
5 Describe the most significant changes and developments which have taken place within the home help setting over the past five years.
6 The half-yearly predictions indicate that your home help budget will exceed the original estimate provision by 10 per cent if left uncorrected. Describe the action needed to be taken to prevent this overspend occurring.
7 You have discovered that a small group of home helps are, outside the time they are normally employed, undertaking additional paid work on behalf of a number of their regular clients. Prepare a memorandum to the Director of Social Services informing him of the position and how you intend to deal with the situation.
8 Most local authorities have benefited under the joint financing arrangements with the former area health authorities. Write fully on:
   (a) how this additional resource has been used to the advantage of the home help service;
   (b) the long-term financial implications facing local authorities as a result of the 'tapering' arrangements.
9 The gradual shift of emphasis from residential to domiciliary care will be strongly felt within the home help service. Describe how the present service will need to change to meet this new development.

PERSONNEL MANAGEMENT

Friday, 18 June 1982
9.30 a.m. to 12.30 p.m.

Answer Question 1, which is compulsory, and THREE other questions
Question 1 carries 40 per cent of the marks
All other questions carry equal marks *Time allowed: 3 hours*

1 *Compulsory question*
   You have recently moved to a new area where little attention has been given to training in the past. You are asked to investigate and recommend ways of improving this situation. Describe what steps you would take:

(a) to establish exactly what training is required;
(b) to set up a systematic training programme;
(c) to organise an induction training programme for new home helps.

2 You suspect that a home help is falsifying her time sheets. Outline the main steps you would take in the course of your investigation and subsequent discipline, bearing in mind the ACAS Code of Practice on Disciplinary Procedures (1977).

3 'Some interviewers would obtain better results by sticking a pin in the list of candidates.' Discuss how the interview can be made as effective as possible in the recruitment and selection procedure.

4 Outline the principles of job evaluation and discuss the advantages and limitations of the technique.

5 Drawing on your own observations at work, describe an episode or a practice which demonstrates good personnel management in action. Give reasons for your choice.

6 Discuss the measures employed in your authority to assist in the supervision of a dispersed labour force, suggesting any improvements that could be made.

7 It has been suggested that people will work harder if you pay them more money. What other factors affect the motivation of people to work?

8 What role should home help organisers have in regard to the safety and health of their employees?

9 Discuss the advantages and disadvantages for management if the home helps wish to join a trade union.

10 Discuss the main points to be noted when conducting a counselling interview. How would you answer criticism that you were 'meddling' in the private lives of your staff?

SOCIAL ADMINISTRATION

Friday, 18 June 1982
2.00 p.m. to 5.00 p.m.

Answer FOUR questions
All questions carry equal marks   *Time allowed: 3 hours*

1 What effects have shortages of resources had on the functioning of the various Welfare State services since the mid-1970s?

2 Do social security provisions aim significantly to reduce inequalities of living standards between those in work and not in work, or merely to provide a basic minimum standard?

3 To what extent should local authority housing policies take account of the needs of special groups such as the elderly and disabled and young single people?

4 Discuss those problems experienced by families on which social policy has focused in recent years. Should State intervention in, and support for, families be increased?

5 Assess the work of social services departments in the field of the care of the elderly. What developments would you anticipate in this field in the future?

6 What do you consider to be the main strengths and weaknesses of using the home help service to prevent some children being taken into care?

7 What problems can arise when workers from different professional groups attempt to work together? Discuss ways in which they can be overcome.

8 Recent thinking in the personal social services has moved in favour of an extreme form of social worker decentralisation known as 'patch-work'. Assess the advantages and disadvantages of this system.

9 How would you describe the function of the domiciliary services within the context of policies of community care?

10 What modifications of the 'Seebohm philosophy' have occurred in practice since the report of 1968 and the Social Services Act of 1970?

References

Amos, G. (1975) *Going Home*. Liverpool: Age Concern.

Andersen, B. R. (1981) *Economic Aspects of Home Help Services*. Copenhagen: Local Government Research Institute on Public Administration and Finance.

Ashdown, M. and Brown, S. (1953) *Social Service and Mental Health*. London: Routledge and Kegan Paul.

Asher, R. A. (1947) Quoted by Barton, R. in *Institutional Neurosis* (1959), 14. Bristol: Wright.

Association of Directors of Social Services (1982) *The Role and Tasks of Social Workers*. Newcastle-upon-Tyne: ADSS.

Association of Municipal Corporations (1960) *Municipal Review Supplement*.

Avon Social Services Department (1980) *Admissions to Homes for the Elderly*. Bristol: Avon County Council.

—— (1982) *Care and Commitment*. Bristol: Avon County Council.

Baert, A. E. (1981) Why do we need alternatives? In *Alternatives to Mental Hospitals*. Report of a European Workshop. London: Mind.

Barclay Report (1982) *Social Workers, their Role and Tasks*. London: Bedford Square Press.

Barton, R. (1959) *Institutional Neurosis*. Bristol: Wright.

Basaglia, F. (1981) Crisis Intervention, Treatment and Rehabilitation. In *Alternatives to Mental Hospitals*. Report of a European Workshop. London: Mind.

Beresford, P. (1982) A Service for Clients. In Philpot, T. (ed.) *A New Direction for Social Work?* London: IPC.

Bessell, R. (1982) Devising an Organisational Structure. In Philpot, T. (ed.) *A New Direction for Social Work?* London: IPC.

Beveridge, W. (1942) *Social Insurance and Allied Services*. Cmd 6404. London: HMSO.

Birch Report (1976) *Working Party on Manpower and Training for the Social Services*. London: DHSS.

Bond, M. (1982) *Women's Work in a Woman's World*. Bristol: School of Advanced Urban Studies.

Booth, C. (1889) *Labour and Life of the People*, Vol. 1: *East London*. London: Williams and Norgate.

Brocklehurst, J. (1978) Ageing and Health. In David Hobman (ed.) *The Social Challenge of Ageing*. London: Croom Helm.

Central Personal Social Services Advisory Committee (1976) *The Needs of Clients and the Role and Responsibilities of Home Helps*. Interim Report of the Sub-Committee on the Home Help Service. Belfast: CPSSAC.

—— (1978) *Administration and Organisation of the Home Help Service*. Second Interim Report of the Sub-Committee on the Home Help Service. Belfast: CPSSAC.

—— (1981) *Recruitment and Training of Home Helps*. Third Interim Report of the Sub-Committee on the Home Help Service. Belfast: CPSSAC.

Cheshire Social Services Department (1980) *Home Help Services in Cheshire*. Chester: Cheshire County Council.

Commission for Local Administration in England and the Representative Body for England (1978) *Complaints Procedures*. London: Representative Body.

Continuing Care Project (1979a) *Home from Hospital: Questions and Answers*. Birmingham: CCP.

—— (1979b) *Communications and Home Care for Patients from Hospital*. Birmingham: CCP.

Davies, B. (1981) Strategic Goals and Piecemeal Innovations: Adjusting to the New Balance of Needs and Resources. In Goldberg, E. M. and Hatch, S. (eds) *A New Look at the Personal Social Services*. London: Policy Studies Institute.

Davis, M. M. (1977) *Homemaker-Home Health Aide Services: A Vital Component in Protective Services for the Elderly*. New York: National HomeCaring Council.

DHSS (1970) *The Future Structure of the National Health Service*. London: HMSO.

—— (1973) *Review of the Home Help Service in England*. London: DHSS.

—— (1976) *A Lifestyle for the Elderly*. London: HMSO.

—— (1977) *Background Paper – Conference on the Elderly*. London: DHSS.

—— (1981a) *Care in the Community*. London: DHSS.

—— (1981b) *Community Care*. London: DHSS.

Dexter, M. (1981) *Home Help Service as a Resource in Somatic Outpatient Care*. Bristol: Avon County Council.

Ferlie, E. (1980) *Directory of Initiatives in Community Care for the Elderly*. Canterbury: University of Kent.

Finer Report (1974) *Report of the Committee on One Parent Families*. London: HMSO.

Flynn, J. A. (1982) Aides for the Elderly. *Health and Social Service Journal* 29 April: 534.

Gibson, R. (1973) In *Care of the Dying*. Proceedings of a National Symposium. London: HMSO.

Gilliand, P. (1977) Trends and Perspectives of Home Help. Propositions for a Policy of Quality of Social Life. In *Current Challenges in the Home Help Services*. Report of Fifth International Congress. Montreux: Swiss Organisation of Home Help Services.

Goldberg, E. M. and Connelly, N. (1982) *The Effectiveness of Social Care for the Elderly*. London: Heinemann.

Gwynne, D. (1980) *Research and Policy-making in the Home Help Service*. Conference Report. Carlisle: Social Services Research Group.

Gwynne, D. and Fean, C. (1978) *The Home Help Service in Cumbria*. Carlisle: Cumbria Social Services Department.

Hamer, A. L. E. (1962) The History of the Home Help Service and its Future. *Journal of the Institute of Home Help Organisers* 10 (18).

Harbert, W. B. (1978) Wanted: A Policy for the Elderly. *Social Work Service* 16.

Harris, A. (1968) *Social Welfare for the Elderly*. London: HMSO.

Harvard Davis Report (1971) *The Organisation of Group Practice*. London: HMSO.

Havighurst, R. (1978) Ageing in Western Societies. In David Hobman (ed.) *The Social Challenge of Ageing*. London: Croom Helm.

Hedley, R. and Norman, A. (1982) *Home Help: Key Issues in Service Provision*. London: Centre for Policy on Ageing.

Hey, A. (1977) *Report of Study Day November 1976*. London: National Council of Home Help Services.

Holford, J. M. (1973) Terminal Care. In *Care of the Dying*. Proceedings of a National Symposium. London: HMSO.

Hunt, A. (1970) *The Home Help Service in England and Wales*. London: HMSO.

—— (1978) *The Elderly at Home*. London: HMSO.

Hyman, M. (1980) *The Home Help Service*. London: Redbridge Social Services Department.

Institute of Home Help Organisers (1954) *The Home Help Organiser* 5 (2).
—— (1958a) *The Training of Home Helps*. Correspondence course. London: IHHO.
—— (1958b) *Journal of the Institute of Home Help Organisers* 7 (14).
—— (1958c) *Journal of the Institute of Home Help Organisers* 6 (12).
—— (1975) *Training of Home Helps*. London: IHHO.
Jay Report (1979) *Report of the Committee of Enquiry into Mental Handicap Nursing and Care*. London: HMSO.
Joint Memorandum of Association of Municipal Corporations and County Councils Association to the National Assistance Board (1951) London: AMC and CCA.
Jonas, C. (1975) *Report on International Seminar held in Frankfurt*. London: National Council of Home Help Services.
Judge, K., Ferlie, E. and Smith, J. (1982) *Charging for Home Help Service*. London: Policy Studies Institute.
Kemm, R. (1977) Synthesis of the Workshop Reports. In *Current Challenges in the Home Help Services*. Report of Fifth International Congress. Montreux: Swiss Organisation of Home Help Services.
Kerstell, T. and Unge, C. (1981) *Home Help Educational Problems*. Stockholm: National Board of Health and Welfare.
Kilbrandon Committee (1964) *Report of the Committee on Children and Young Persons (Scotland)*. Edinburgh: HMSO.
Kivela, Sirkka-Liisa (1981) *Social and Health Service Car for Out-patient Care*. Helsinki: Finnish National Committee of the International Council of Home Help Services.
Leslie, M. (1972) *Through Changing Scenes*. Beaconsfield: Mary Leslie.
Local Government Training Board (1978) *Training of Home Helps*. Luton: LGTB.
London Boroughs Home Help Services Managers Group (1978) *London's Home Help Service. A Review of the Organisation and Practice of the Home Help Service in the London Boroughs. First Report*. London: LBHHSMG.
McCleary, G. F. (1935) *The Maternity and Child Welfare Movement*. Quoted by McEwan, M. in *Health Visiting* (1951). London: Faber and Faber.
McGrath, M. and Hadley, R. (1981) Evaluating Patch-based Social Services Teams: A Pilot Study. In Goldberg, E. M. and Connelly, N. (eds) *Evaluating Research in Social Care*. London: Heinemann.
Majuri, R. (1981) *Home Help Services as a Special Resource to Multi-Problem Families*. Helsinki: National Board of Social Welfare.
Mayumi, M. (1962) Home Help Service within Industry in Japan. *Journal of the Institute of Home Help Organisers* 11 (21).

National Association of Home Help Organisers (1949a) *The Home Help Organiser* 1 (6).

—— (1949b) *The Home Help Organiser* 1 (9).

—— (1952) *Home Help and the Nations. Report of First International Conference on the Home Help Service*. London: NAHHO.

National Board of Health and Welfare (1981) *Social Rehabilitation of the Multi-Handicapped*. Stockholm: NBHW.

National Council for Homemaker–Home Health Aide Services (1981) *Home Help Services as a Resource in Psychiatric Outpatient Care*. New York: NCHHHAS.

National Council of Home Help Services (1975) *Report on Questionnaire relating to Scales of Allowances and Charges made for Home Help Service*. London: NCHHS.

—— (1976) *Conference Papers on Study Day*. London: NCHHS.

—— (1979) *Home Help Services in Great Britain*. London: NCHHS.

—— (1981) *Health and Safety*. London: NCHHS.

Nusberg, C. (1981) Programmes and Services for the Elderly in Industrialised Countries. In Hobman, D. (ed.) *The Impact of Ageing*. London: Croom Helm.

Ogilvie, G. (1951) Overseas Visitors. *The Home-Help Organiser* 3 (26).

Parker, R. (1980) Policies, Presumptions and Prospects in Charging for the Social Services. In Judge, K. (ed.) *Pricing the Social Services*. London: Macmillan.

—— (1981) Tending and Social Policy. In Goldberg, E. M. and Hatch, S. (eds) *A New Look at the Personal Social Services*. London: Policy Studies Institute.

Parsloe, P. (1981) *Social Services Area Teams*. London: Allen and Unwin.

Pearce Report (1974) *Training for Organisers of Home Help and Other Supportive Domiciliary Services*. London: CCETSW and LGTB.

Personal Social Services Council (1976) *Complaints Procedures in the Personal Social Services*. London: PSSC.

Quelsh, K. (1981) A Choice to Stay at Home. *Health and Social Service Journal* 29 October: 1336–8.

Redcliffe-Maud Committee (1974) *Conduct in Local Government*. London: HMSO.

Robens Committee (1972) *Safety and Health at Work*. London: HMSO.

Rowbottom, R., Hey, A., and Billis, D. (1978) *Social Services Departments Developing Patterns of Work and Organisation*. London: Heinemann.

Rowlings, C. (1981) *Social Work with Elderly People*. London: Allen and Unwin.

Rowntree, B. (1901) *Poverty – A Study of Town Life*. London:

Macmillan.

Scottish Education Department, Scottish Home and Health Department (1966) *Social Work and the Community*. Edinburgh: HMSO.

Seebohm Committee (1968) *Report of the Committee on Local Authority and Allied Personal Social Services*. London: HMSO.

Simey, M. (1951) *Charitable Effort in Liverpool in the Nineteenth Century*. Liverpool University Press.

Somerset Social Services Department (1980) *Home Care Survey*. Taunton: Somerset County Council.

Stevenson, O. (1977) *Social Work Research Project. Final Report*. Universities of Aberdeen and Keele. Quoted in CPSSAC (1978).

Stockholm Social Welfare Board (1980) Descriptions of Situations where Home Helps have to lift Patients. In *Information Bulletin* 18. Utrecht: International Council of Home Help Services.

—— (1981) *Caring for One Another*. Stockholm: SSWB.

Supplementary Benefits Commission (1980) *Notes and News* July (17).

Swedish Post Office (1981) *Social Services provided by Rural Postmen in Sweden*. Stockholm: SPO.

Thompson, C. G. K. (1964) Ideas for Reshaping the Local Health Services. *The Municipal Journal* 10 January: 87.

Tizard, J. and Grad, J. C. (1961) *Maudsley Monograph* 7. London: Maudsley Hospital.

Ward, M. (1960) The Hospital Almoner and General Practitioner. *Case Conference* 7 (5).

West Sussex County Council (1981) *Home Help Charges*. Chichester: WSCC.

White, D. T. (1975) *Conference Report*. London: Institute of Home Help Organisers.

Wilkes, E. (1973) In *Care of the Dying*. Proceedings of a National Symposium. London: HMSO.

Younghusband Report (1959) *Report of the Working Party on Social Workers in the Local Authority, Health and Welfare Services*. London: HMSO.

Index

Grad, J. C., 83
group practices, 50
Gwynne, D., 125, 158

Hadley, R., 170
Hamer, A. L. E., 187
handicapped, the, 197
'handywomen', 8
Harbert, W. B., 90
Harris, A., 138
Harvard Davis Report (1971), 50, 81
health and safety, 106–10
Health and Safety at Work Act (1974), 106, 107
health service, the, 174, 198
health visitors, 6
Hedley, R., 169
Hey, A., 56, 172–73
Hill, Octavia, 6
Holford, J. M., 30
home help/client match, 123
home help/client ratios, 60
home help/client relationship, 34–5
home help/organiser ratios, 60, 110
home help organisers: administrative functions of, 152; appointment of, 201–02; and assessment, 115–16; and home helps, 24–5, 160–61; and legislation, 110–11; pay of, 105; responsibilities of, 95; role of, 79, 82–3, 173–74; and safety, 108; training of, 185–93
home help service: definition of, 66; growth of, 1949–53, 13; international development of, 62–9; and management models, 56–61; numbers employed in, 32, 49, 67, 210–11; number of managerial posts in, 163; objectives of, 78–9; and other caring services, 80–3, 147; privatisation of, 199; professional aspects of management of, 146–49; public image of, 36; reorganisations of, 46–50; and residential care, 90–1; in south-west, 85, 86; speed of response of, 149; studies of effectiveness of, 88–9; trends in allocation of, 88; unique problems of, 172
home help stamps, 142

home helps: and assessment, 123–24; duties appropriate to, 212–13; personal burden on, 161–62; tasks undertaken by, 32–4; training for, 178–85; working conditions of, 203–06
homemakers, 72–7
hospice movement, 31
hospitals: care on leaving, 30, 40, 81–2, 176; death in, 30–1; and free home care services, 134–35; and length of stay in, 26; and local health authorities, 46–7
hourly charges, 140
housing, 51
housing estates, 20
Hulth, M., 68
Hunt, A., 21, 35, 89, 135–36, 138–39, 140, 154, 155, 160
hygiene, 3, 181
Hyman, M., 141

Iceland, 67
infant mortality, 8, 62
informal carers, 29–31
in-service training, 151, 193
Institute of Home Help Organisers, 13–14, 37–8, 133, 179, 182, 185, 186, 187, 188, 190, 207
'institutional neurosis', 24
institutionalisation, 24–5
institutions, care in, 24–9
insurance, 198
integrated domiciliary care, experiments in, 170–71
intensified family help, 74–7
intensity, as a technical term, 84–5, 89–90, 93
international conferences, 199–200
International Congress of Home Help Services (1981), 20, 68, 72
International Council of Home Help Services, 14, 62, 66, 67, 68, 109, 200
inter-professional rivalry, 169
Israel, 64, 65–6
Italy, 27, 63
itemised pay statement, 99–100

Japan, 64, 66, 162
jargon words, 83